PRAISE FOR *BEYOND THE WALLS*

"Dr. Neuwirth is one of the brightest and most constructive leaders and commentators in healthcare. He has an incredible perspective on healthcare and a positive humanistic viewpoint. It's people like Zeev Neuwirth who give me hope that we can solve the daunting challenges in caring for 330 million Americans whose population is growing and aging."

—Scott Becker, publisher, Becker's Healthcare

"Zeev is a foremost thinker on the American healthcare system. This book outlines the major issues and considerations driving better health outcomes and experience at lower costs. A must-read for anyone interested in value-based care in the US now and in the future."

—Patrick Conway, MD, CEO of Care Solutions, Optum

"Zeev Neuwirth has given the world a gift. This new work provides us with a master view of what works and how things need to be changed in healthcare. It shines a light on proven concepts as well as some of the courageous leaders who are working to change things for the better."

—Michellene Davis, Esq., president and CEO, National Medical Fellowships, Inc.

"In *Beyond the Walls*, Zeev shares poignant examples of how healthcare is being transformed and the profound benefits to patients and providers. I see this book as a wake-up call for policy makers and healthcare leaders—to recognize the importance of getting beyond the walls and to reduce the risks and barriers that our healthcare system imposes on those who seek to rehumanize it."

—Sean Duffy, CEO and cofounder, Omada Health

"The American healthcare system needs to change. We all know that. What we need is fresh thinking and new solutions. In *Beyond the Walls*, Dr. Neuwirth shares his wisdom, empathy, and solutions on how to move beyond the literal, conceptual, and systemic walls of the past. This book should be read by every decision maker and policy maker in American healthcare."

—Joseph J. Fifer, CPA, FHFMA; president and CEO, Healthcare Financial Management Association

"*Beyond the Walls* is a groundbreaking analysis and brilliantly curated guide for the much-needed reform in our healthcare industry. It should be read by anyone who wants to be part of the solution and not part of the problem."

—Ruby Gadelrab, CEO and founder, MDisrupt

"Too many books about healthcare talk about how we tear down the walls. Zeev Neuwirth's new book takes the landmark approach of creating a better system. Read this book if you want to go beyond what's wrong with American healthcare and want to be optimistic about where it can go!"

—Steve Klasko, MD, MBA, former president and CEO, Thomas Jefferson University and Jefferson Health

"Dr. Neuwirth provides a fascinating analysis of the current state of American healthcare and offers practical solutions for how to transcend its limitations. This book is an essential read, and I highly recommend it to anyone who wants to contribute to the future of our nation's healthcare system."

—Hal Paz, MD, CEO, Stony Brook Medicine; executive vice president for Health Sciences, Stony Brook University

"Zeev Neuwirth has a remarkable ability to take complex healthcare changes and make them actionable. Rather than just lamenting about all that is wrong, he focuses on how people are making medical care right. And as a result, he lights a path to better health for America's future."

—Robert Pearl, MD, former CEO, The Permanente Medical Group; professor, Stanford University Schools of Business

"Very few people exhibit Zeev's penetrating vision into our healthcare system. His insistence on getting to the 'why' instead of just reporting on the 'what' is invaluable to anyone attempting to navigate the healthcare industry."

—Roy Schoenberg, CEO and cofounder, Amwell

"Dr. Zeev Neuwirth's insightful reflections offer professional and historical perspectives on why American healthcare operates the way it does. It's an important read for anyone working to make a difference in our system."

—The Honorable David J. Shulkin, MD, Ninth Secretary, US Department of Veterans Affairs

"Dr. Neuwirth challenges us to empower health consumers. He urges us not to settle for incremental changes that perpetuate the status quo but to dismantle the barriers that have restricted innovation and disruption. *Beyond the Walls* is a call to action to bring humanity back into our healthcare system."

—Glen Tullman, CEO, Transcarent & Medicine

"Dr. Neuwirth's latest book presents practical approaches to transform the broken American healthcare system. The examples he shares propel us to take collective actions that go beyond the same old ways of doing things. It is an engaging and energizing read that speaks to the truth-seeker in all of us."

—Sara Vaezy, chief strategy and digital officer, Providence

BEYOND THE WALLS

Zeev E. Neuwirth, MD

BEYOND THE WALLS

Megatrends, Movements, and Market Disruptors
TRANSFORMING AMERICAN HEALTHCARE

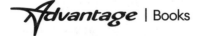 | Books

Published by Advantage Books, Charleston, South Carolina.
An imprint of Advantage Media.

ADVANTAGE is a registered trademark, and the Advantage colophon is a trademark of Advantage Media Group, Inc.

Printed in the United States of America.

10 9 8 7 6 5 4 3 2 1

ISBN: 978-1-64225-382-5 (Hardcover)
ISBN: 978-1-64225-641-3 (eBook)

Library of Congress Control Number: 2023910154

Book design by Megan Elger.

This publication is designed to provide accurate and authoritative information in regard to the subject matter covered. It is sold with the understanding that the publisher is not engaged in rendering legal, accounting, or other professional services. If legal advice or other expert assistance is required, the services of a competent professional person should be sought.

Advantage Books is an imprint of Advantage Media Group. Advantage Media helps busy entrepreneurs, CEOs, and leaders write and publish a book to grow their business and become the authority in their field. Advantage authors comprise an exclusive community of industry professionals, idea-makers, and thought leaders. For more information go to **advantagemedia.com**.

To healthcare professionals and the staff
who directly and indirectly support patient care.
I appreciate the challenging and important nature
of the work you do. My intent with this book is to
advance a healthcare system that is better for all of us
and more supportive of your efforts.

CONTENTS

PART III: MARKET DISRUPTORS

HITTING THE WALLS

I BEGAN "HITTING THE WALL" three decades ago. I realized very early on in my training that the way we were delivering healthcare was decidedly suboptimal in many ways. I had entered into a system that was demoralizing to patients, to their families, and to those who provided care. I knew I needed to do something about it, not just to make it better but also to make it fundamentally different—to make it, for lack of a better term, *humanistic*. To be clear, I'm not referring to the aspirations or actions of the professionals who provide care. My observation is that the people working within healthcare have an intrinsic motivation to serve others. Instead, the problem was, and continues to be, the system of healthcare itself. Given that realization, my overarching mission became clear—to transform the healthcare delivery system. Three decades later, this has remained my aim, and it's guided me throughout my entire career. Looking back, I recall many moments that have propelled and fueled this mission. But there were three relatively recent moments that set me on a different and unanticipated trajectory. I think about these as my "matrix moments."

If you're a fan of the classic 1999 sci-fi movie *The Matrix*, you know what I'm talking about. For those who haven't seen it, the plot involves a computer hacker named Neo who has a troubling intuitive sense that his day-to-day reality isn't quite right—it's not as it appears to be. As Neo's suspicions grow, he meets a mysterious man named Morpheus, who addresses Neo's disorientation and later becomes his guide and mentor. I'm going to share a snippet from the movie because I believe that Morpheus's message is likely the reason you're reading these pages.

> *Let me tell you why you're here. You're here because you know something. What you know you can't explain, but you feel it. You've felt it your entire life, that there's something wrong.... You don't know what it is, but it's there.... It is this feeling that has brought you to me.*

In 2014 my mother, Ruth, went into the hospital for an elective hip surgery. She was in relatively good health at the age of seventy-four but ended up dying from a bacterial infection and the septic shock that ensued. In the healthcare quality and safety field, what led to her death is termed a "hospital-acquired condition," or HAC. The tragedy is that her death was easily preventable if the providers and staff in that hospital had followed well-established safety protocols. The literature on healthcare safety informs us that most preventable deaths actually arise from a series of errors. My mother's case was textbook in this regard. The harsh irony is that the very system I had served in my entire professional life had failed my mother and my family, just as it fails hundreds of other individuals and families every single day. For me, this failure was no longer an abstract statistic or professional observation. The loss of my mother hit me hard on such a deep and personal level that I was forever changed. In addition to the grief I felt, I was overwhelmed by the guilt of not being able to save my mother's life. I've played the experience over and over again in my head, and I know there were opportunities I missed that might have altered the course of events. This was my first matrix moment.

My second matrix moment occurred within a year of my mother's death. It was what I describe as a "groundhog day" experience. For those of you who've seen the movie *Groundhog Day*, you'll recall that the main character is forced to relive the same day over and over again. As a healthcare executive, I felt like I was reliving the same meetings over and over again—a sentiment I've heard expressed by healthcare executives and physicians across the country. One meeting in particular left me with an unforgettable visceral feeling. We were discussing the issue of access—the weeks of waiting time our patients were experiencing in order to see a physician—a pervasive and worsening problem within our healthcare system. We were reviewing some tactics to address this problem when I was struck by the memory of a meeting I had with these same physicians and administrators a few years prior, discussing the same problem, reviewing the same exact solutions. It was as if we were stuck in some sort of time warp. Then my mind flashed to another meeting. This one had taken place a whole decade earlier in a different organization, with a different set of doctors and administrators. But again, we were focused on the exact same problem and a similar set of solutions. Little to nothing had fundamentally changed in over a decade. This realization was disconcerting, to say the least. It left me with a pit in my stomach and with a drive in my heart to do something about it. That sensibility has never left me.

My third matrix moment involved another sad and unexpected personal loss. A close physician colleague and friend committed suicide. He was also my primary care doctor, so our relationship ran deep. As with my mother's death, an all-too-common statistic had now become a personal trauma. This third event was a tipping point. I remember sitting at my desk in my home study on an early Saturday morning. I was catching up with emails and wrapping up some work left over from the week when I received the short text telling me my friend was gone. I'll never forget that text or that moment. I sat there, transfixed, staring at the floor beneath my feet. In that moment, I could sense myself descending into guilt, then depression, and then despair. Similar to the experience with my mother, I wondered if there was something I could have done to prevent my friend's death. After a while, my guilt, fear, and doubt turned into anger. I gritted my teeth and shook my head slowly from side to side. "No," I said to myself silently. "No."

I, once again, felt like Neo in *The Matrix* at that moment when Morpheus offers him a choice.

> *This is your last chance. After this, there is no turning back. You take the blue pill—the story ends, you wake up in your bed and believe whatever you want to believe. You take the red pill—you stay in Wonderland, and I show you how deep the rabbit hole goes. Remember, all I'm offering is the truth—nothing more.*

At that moment—my third matrix moment—I decided to take the "red pill." Like Neo, I felt the need to escape the artificial and opaque reality that I was living in. Like Neo, I couldn't go back, and I couldn't pretend any longer. Like Neo, I wanted to know the truth that I couldn't see, in my case, behind the confusing complexities of our healthcare system and beyond the walls of my present discernment. And like Neo, I wanted to create a new and more humanistic reality, in my case, within our healthcare system.

So I began this journey with a goal—to avoid mindlessly perpetuating the current perverse shortcomings and constraints of our healthcare system. I set out to train myself to perceive the realities and to identify the hopeful possibilities that were emerging. I wanted genuine progress. I wanted to go beyond the walls. As I ventured farther and farther outside of the confines of traditional healthcare, I began to rekindle my belief that we deserve a better healthcare system and, importantly, to believe that we can make that the dominant reality.

After experiencing those matrix moments, I began to seek out my own Morpheus-like figures—unconventional, courageous guides who could introduce me to this new reality. I began to connect with bold leaders and entrepreneurs who had also taken the "red pill." Many of them were working outside of the legacy system, but all of them were transcending the constraining walls of the past. I sought out visionary leaders who were crafting workable, game-changing solutions that seemed long overdue.

Several years ago, in 2016, I began recording my conversations—the in-depth interviews with these transformational leaders. I studied the transcripts looking for patterns, and I began sharing my learnings with colleagues. At the urging of peers, I began posting these interviews in the form of a podcast, *Creating a New Healthcare*, which I've hosted since 2017. At this point in time, I've recorded over three hundred in-depth interviews and shared nearly half of them. These formal interviews, plus the thousands of other conversations I've had as a healthcare executive over the past seventeen years, form the basis for much of what I'll share in this book. It's important to understand that what's offered in this book is derived from individuals and organizations that are actually changing healthcare. While I truly appreciate theory and thought leadership, like many of you, I'm from the "show me" state. I am, at heart, an empiricist. I believe what I can see to be working.

The story I've just shared with you is my personal and professional story. But the story that unfolds within this book is a story about American healthcare. And while my overarching approach is to identify, appreciate, and highlight what's right in American healthcare, I feel it's important to take a moment to recognize the stark and irrefutable reality that, as it's currently organized, our healthcare system has hit the wall. In the hundreds of interviews I've conducted with healthcare experts and leaders over the past seven years, there is not one—*not one*—who believes that our healthcare system is serving the needs of the American people and not one who believes that our healthcare system is economically sustainable. There is an abundance of research studies, reports, and books that document and substantiate these claims. So instead of further elaborating on these points, I'm going to focus our attention on how to transcend the system and get beyond its limitations.

In *Beyond the Walls*, I am not going to dwell on what's wrong with American healthcare. Instead, I'm going to delve into what's right. The stories I've chronicled in these pages are inspiring, real-life transformations that we need to adopt and spread. As you'll witness, we have begun to break free of the spiraling negativity and inertia of the past. I've experienced it, and I feel compelled to share this increasingly positive perspective. It is a countertheme in an industry that has frustrated, angered, and even harmed Americans for decades.

Let's now discover together just what lies "beyond the walls."

I'm often asked how I select my podcast interviewees. There are a number of criteria I use, which include:

1. Leaders who have built or created something unique, or who have had a significant positive impact on American healthcare delivery.

2. Leaders who have "stood up and stepped out." By that, I mean that they have taken a divergent perspective and acted upon it, putting their time, energy, reputation, resources, and even their careers on the line.

3. Leaders who have exhibited the courage and commitment to a cause they believe to be beyond their own financial or personal gain.

4. Leaders who are painfully frustrated with the status quo and want to do more than complain.

5. Leaders who are reframing healthcare—a road map for which I've shared in the supplement to this book.

6. Leaders who have experienced firsthand and in a very personal way the unintended harm that our system can cause.

INTRODUCTION
BEYOND THE WALLS

WHEN I FIRST STARTED drafting this book, the working title was *The Future of Healthcare Is Here and Now*. It captured much of what I had been writing about—the transformations in healthcare that were already occurring and my hope that we could then resource, emulate, and spread them. But deep down, I knew that the title was not quite right. One night I awoke from sleep, triggered by something I remembered from a book I had read a year or two earlier. I couldn't remember the title or the author, but I knew the metaphor that I was looking for. So I searched every bookshelf and drawer in our home and finally found the book. It was titled *The Innovation Stack* and was written by a brilliantly successful serial entrepreneur, Jim McKelvey.[1] I immediately turned to a few lines in the first chapter where Jim defines the "entrepreneurial" persona. Using criteria similar to those I used in selecting the individuals featured in this book, Jim describes an entrepreneur as "a special type of person: a risk taker who reshaped an industry through innovation ... revolutionaries ... rebels, explorers, and people driven by more than just profit or even common sense."[2]

---

1   Jim McKelvey, *The Innovation Stack: Building an Unbeatable Business One Crazy Idea at a Time* (New York: Portfolio, 2020).

2   McKelvey, *The Innovation Stack*, 4.

A couple of pages further into the chapter, Jim has a section titled "The Walled City." This was the metaphor and image that woke me up from my sleep. Here's what he writes:

> Draw a giant circle around everything humankind knows.... [P]icture that circle as a physical border, like the wall around an ancient city. Medieval Edinburgh was such a city, with a giant stone wall protecting and confining the citizens inside.... As literally crappy as life in the city was, it was preferable to the wilderness outside. But not for everyone. Some people left the city. Maybe they looked over the wall and asked, "What can I do out there?"... Beyond the wall there were no laws, except for those of nature. And because nature uses capital punishment to enforce basically everything, the price of failure is steep.... If you stay within this metaphorical wall, you are a sane businessperson. If you leave the world of the known, you are an entrepreneur or a corpse.... It is these crazy entrepreneurs and their perfect problems that bring us the future.[3]

And by "perfect problem," he means, "A perfect problem has a solution, but not a solution that exists yet. There are countless problems in the world; many of them have existing solutions while others lie beyond our current capabilities. But between these two extremes lie some problems that we can solve if we invent a new way."[4]

Jim's perfect problem echoes the career framing observation of Clayton Christensen, the renowned Harvard Business School professor, who wrote, "When the business world encounters an intractable management problem, it's a sign that business executives and scholars are getting something wrong—that there isn't yet a satisfactory theory for what's causing the problem, and under what circum-

---

3   McKelvey, *The Innovation Stack*, 8–10.

4   McKelvey, *The Innovation Stack*, 7.

stance it can be overcome."[5] It's obvious to me that we are precisely in this situation in American healthcare and have been for decades. If the problem were fixable within our current framework, it would have been solved by now. It is clear that healthcare is one of those problems that requires us to invent a new way. Those passages from Jim's book also made clear to me that the metaphor and the title I had been looking for was "beyond the walls." It captures the mindset, the spirit, and the actions of the trailblazing leaders and organizations portrayed in this book.

As this idea relates to healthcare entrepreneurs, there are three beliefs I hold that build upon Jim's elegant metaphor. First, I believe that there are many people working within the legacy healthcare system who have the same courageous spirit and impact as those who venture into the world of start-ups. Second, my belief is that progress is made not just by the isolated entrepreneurial activities outside the walls but also by those advances being brought back and forth over the walls to be shared, integrated, and spread. The key point here is not to focus on the wall but to transcend it, whether to leap over it or to render it permeable. Third, while "the walls" are a metaphor, the first section of this book actually illustrates how healthcare today is getting beyond the literal concrete walls of hospitals and clinics.

BEYOND THE WALLS: THE THREE DOMAINS

As I began to adopt the 'beyond the walls' metaphor, I noticed that each section of this book described a different perspective on the metaphor. This unexpected synchronicity further cemented my intuition that what we need in healthcare is *a 'beyond the walls' movement*. The three

---

5   MIT Sloan Management Review, *When Innovation Moves at Digital Speed: Strategies and Tactics to Provoke, Sustain, and Defend Innovation in Today's Unsettled Markets* (Cambridge: MIT Press, 2019), 140.

domains of 'beyond the walls' are transcendence of the walls at a (1) concrete or literal level, (2) a conceptual level, and (3) a systemic level. To be clear, **all three domains are interconnected** and **all three are necessary** if we are to get "beyond the walls."

Part I of this book is titled "Megatrends." This section corresponds to the first domain of 'beyond the walls'—the transposition of healthcare beyond the walls of brick-and-mortar hospitals, emergency departments, urgent care centers, lab testing centers, primary and specialty care clinics, and nursing homes. In the foreseeable future, there will continue to be a need for these centralized facilities. However, we are moving to a both/and situation, a hybrid approach of in-person, virtual, and automated care. Part II is titled "Movements," which I would characterize as *humanistic* movements. This second section corresponds to the transcendence of healthcare beyond the *conceptual* walls, liberating ourselves from dogmatic and restrictive thinking. This requires us to reframe healthcare within new orientations and to redefine the problems in order to create new solutions. Part III is titled "Market Disruptors" and illustrates the systemic transcendence beyond the walls of our healthcare system. Platforms, titanic disruptors, and strategic partnerships are all changes at the system level. They encompass digital capabilities and emerging communication channels, new business models and operational infrastructures, novel contractual collaborations, and more collaborative governorship structures.

THE 'BEYOND THE WALLS' MOVEMENT IS ALREADY HAPPENING

These three perspectives of the 'beyond the walls' metapohor involve fundamental changes to the entire system of American healthcare as we've known it. These are not hypothetical or future changes. The

BEYOND THE WALLS

THE THREE DOMAINS

LITERAL

Virtual, Digital &
Automated Care

Point of Need
is Point of Care

Home-Based Care
Ecosystem

CONCEPTUAL

Diversity, Equity
& Inclusion

Non-Clinical
Determinants of
Health

Customized,
Contextual & Whole
Health Care

SYSTEMIC

Platforms

Partnerships,
Collaborations &
Integrations

Payment &
Policy Reform

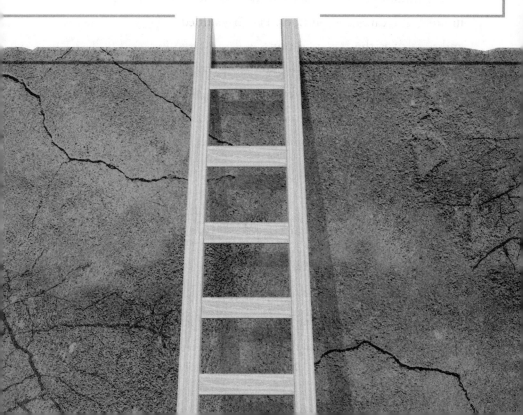

transformations depicted in this book are all about the present. As author William Gibson wrote, "The future is already here. It's just not evenly distributed yet."[6] The reality is that most of the transformative changes described in this book have been going on for years. And these game-changing overhauls are not unique to healthcare. They're connected to a much larger set of transformations that have been taking place over the past few decades in numerous other industries. These industries have all gone through the concrete, conceptual, and systemic 'beyond the walls' transformations that healthcare is currently undergoing. These are seismic revolutions that have radically changed our daily lives.

For example, think about the ways we communicate now—via smart phones and social media channels. On a daily basis, we email, text, blog, and use Teams, Webex, and Zoom. We also use Facebook, LinkedIn, Twitter, TikTok, Instagram, Snapchat, WhatsApp, and YouTube not only to communicate bits of information but also to form and maintain communities. Think about the way we do our banking. When was the last time you waited in line for a teller? Do some of you even know what a bank teller is? And how about the forms of entertainment we now take for granted—an endless set of options, including Netflix, Amazon Prime, Disney Channel, HBO, Hulu, and so on. In the not-too-distant past, if you wanted information, you'd likely head to the library or perhaps open up a hard copy encyclopedia. Now search engines such as Google have become a verb, as in "let me google it." When was the last time you tried to fix something without consulting YouTube? And with the recent advent of machine learning, we are seeing the world of content and analytics being transformed through the power of artificial intelligence (AI), not only providing us with answers but also with productivity—from

---

6   As quoted in the *San Francisco Examiner* by Scott Rosenberg, 1992.

writing documents to creating software code to automating manual labor. Think, too, about the way we book vacations and the way we travel. You can book anything from a mansion to a houseboat to a studio apartment online and instantly. And for those of us who have already converted to electric vehicles, we understand that it's not so much a traditional car that we're sitting in but a highly networked digital platform. Finally, think about the way physical exercise has changed. If you're not tracking some part of your physiology or your activity—steps, calories, heart rate, weight, body fat, energy efficiency—with digital tools, I would be surprised.

Banking, finance, retail, commerce, communication, content, entertainment, travel, and fitness have all been completely transfigured and have substantially changed our daily lives. Now it's healthcare's turn. As I've noted, this transformation is not entirely new to healthcare, and it has become more noticeable. To loosely paraphrase Winston Churchill, we are not at the beginning of this 'beyond the walls' transformation; we are at the end of the beginning and about to enter a much more apparent phase of the 'beyond the walls' era in American healthcare delivery.

HISTORICAL LESSON BEYOND THE WALLS

As I began to create the 'beyond the walls' metaphor, it dawned on me that there were numerous walled cities erected during the Middle Ages. Google them, and you'll quickly see what I'm talking about. In addition to Edinburgh, the ones that immediately come to mind are Paris, London, and Florence. What also comes to mind is the well-known saying that if we don't study history, we'll be condemned to relive it. History teaches us that the walls of these great cities served an important purpose in their time—namely, protection. But over time that purpose was superseded by the need for greater communication, greater connectivity, greater community, and advances in culture and commerce. Maintaining the walls—from the literal to conceptual to systemic levels—became a vulnerability, not a strength. The freer flow and integration of people, ideas, culture, technologies, and trade became critical for the advancement of civilization.

I'm not a historian, and I'm not sure if the great shift from the Dark Ages to the Renaissance was due, in part, to the transcendence of these walls, but I wouldn't doubt it. The larger and more relevant lesson, however, is one that should not be lost on us in healthcare. Our walls were developed for a purpose and a reason that made sense *in their time*. That time is long gone. What we now need is to rapidly get beyond the walls, to embrace the renaissance that is currently underway. The urgency is nothing less than a matter of life and death. My hope is that this book helps further catalyze, inform, and inspire the 'beyond the walls' movement in American healthcare delivery.

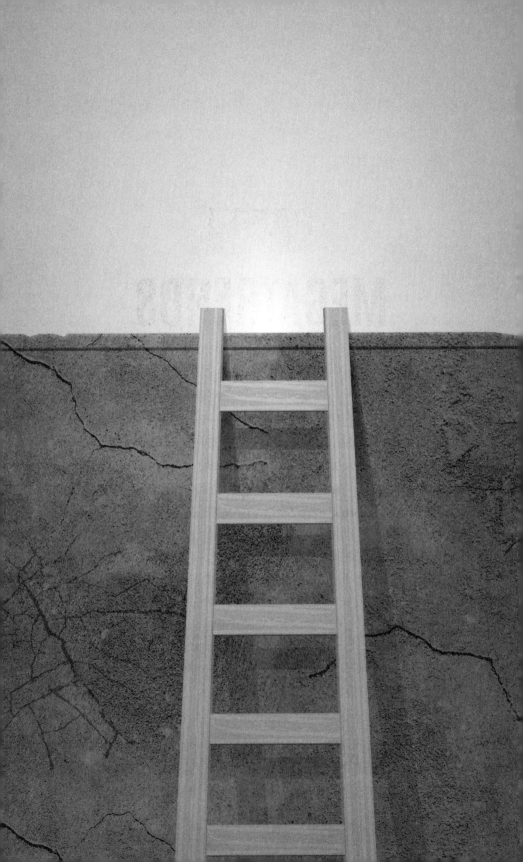

PART I

MEGATRENDS

The industry has become very hungry for reinventing itself through technology and it will happen much faster than any other revolution healthcare has gone through. This one is for the people, and that is why healthcare is going to change faster than we think.
—**Roy Schoenberg, CEO and cofounder, Amwell**

IN PART I, WE WILL TAKE a close look at the transformational healthcare megatrends that have been snowballing within our society. These are powerful forces, poised to permanently change how we experience, receive, and engage in healthcare. These fundamental forces take us beyond the walls of what we've known healthcare delivery to be during the past few decades. In 2021 Andy Jassy, Amazon's CEO, responding to a question in a community-wide meeting, said that ten years from now, the standard experience of seeing a doctor would seem "crazy."[7] I couldn't agree more. I believe we're going to see a major decentralization, disaggregation, and democratization of care, and it's going to happen this decade.

From a 'beyond the walls' perspective, we are witnessing the actual movement of care from within the centralized brick-and-mortar walls of clinics and hospitals to decentralized locations. We are seeing the delivery of care shift to where we live our lives—in our homes, at work, and in our communities. It's a transposition of time, space, and need.

In chapter 1 we'll discuss the digital health revolution, which will be the required technology base that will enable us to transcend the walls. It's akin to a modern-day Gutenberg press but on steroids. That fifteenth-century technology ushered in a new age of enlightenment, as will the twenty-first-century digital revolution that is now upon us. Chapter 2 will illustrate how we are in the midst of a shift in care away from being episodic, intermittent, and reactive to care that is delivered where and when we need it. That's also a transposition of time, space, and need, with the point of need becoming the point of care. In chapter 3, we continue tracking the decentralization of care from the brick-and-mortar hospital to the hospital at home. This trend has been around for years, but with the recent catalytic effect of the COVID-19 pandemic, it's now becoming a mainstay of care delivery. The trend extends beyond acute hospital care to include all aspects of the continuum of care. And as we'll discover, it's not only more convenient, satisfactory, cost-effective, and safer than legacy brick-and-mortar settings; it also opens the door for many of the humanistic movements we'll discuss in part II.

---

7   Eugene Kim and Blake Dodge, "In Leaked Audio, Amazon's CEO Andy Jassy Shares a Bold Vision," *Business Insider*, March 18, 2022, https://www.businessinsider.com/amazon-ceo-andy-jassy-shares-bold-vision-for-healthcare-business-2022-3.

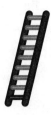

DIGITAL—THE GREAT ENABLER

*The digital revolution is far more significant than
the invention of writing or even of printing.*
–Douglas Engelbart

T rying to describe digital healthcare in a single chapter is like trying to capture moonbeams in your hands. It's an impossible task, given the enormity of the topic and the speed with which the technology and its influence is expanding. From the music and entertainment industries to banking and finance, from telecom to real estate, retail, and travel, entire industries have been radically transformed and vastly improved by digitalization over the past couple of decades. That improvement represents a quantum leap in how we do things and the capabilities we possess. For example, in 2015 only 9.5 percent of Americans used mobile banking as their primary method. Now that adoption is over 40 percent and rapidly growing.[8] The digital real estate provider

---

8 "2021 FDIC National Survey of Unbanked and Underbanked Households," Federal Deposit Insurance Corporation, November 14, 2022, https://www.fdic.gov/analysis/household-survey/.

Zillow had only 54 million unique visitors in 2012. In 2021 that number had grown to 234 million.[9] And according to the Census Bureau, less than 6 percent of all retail sales were e-commerce sales. That number has since jumped to nearly 15 percent.[10]

Digitalization is doing the same for healthcare. First, it's important to define what we mean by digital healthcare. It's not just about virtual telehealth visits, which involve the use of communication channels that allow for care through audio or video exchanges. Digital here refers to the exchange of information, enabling of communication, and efficiency of automation that has been made possible by digital technologies. It encompasses remote physiologic monitoring, automated communications, and real-time alerts. It refers to the data analytics that identify those patients at risk of disease or drug interaction, matching individuals with the right providers, finding geographically convenient clinics, and deploying healthcare products and services personalized to individuals' needs. It refers to the digital analytics and AI-enabled tech that is revolutionizing our diagnostic capabilities, enhancing research, and enabling us to create new medications and therapeutics in unprecedented ways. In this book, "digital" refers to the enabling technologies that are already embedded as a critical component in the delivery of state-of-the-art clinical care in hospitals, in operating rooms, in radiology suites, and in doctor's offices. More than any other single factor, these new abilities are allowing us to completely reframe healthcare delivery. In just a few short years, almost no aspect of healthcare will be possible without digital technology. Digital is "the great enabler" in healthcare.

---

9   "Zillow Statistics," iPropertyManagement, October 12, 2022, https://ipropertyman-agement.com/research/zillow-statistics.

10 "Quarterly Retail E-Commerce Sales 4th Quarter 2022," US Census Bureau News, Washington, DC, February 17, 2023, https://www.census.gov/retail/mrts/www/data/pdf/ec_current.pdf.

OUR ETHER MOMENT

One of the first healthcare entrepreneurs I interviewed about digitization was Sean Duffy. He had already been schooling me about digital health for five years *prior* to our first official 2017 podcast interview. Sean cofounded the digital healthcare platform Omada in 2011 with the aim of merging evidence-based programs with cutting-edge technology to revolutionize the care of chronic disease as we know it. In 2012, when I first met Sean, I had no idea what digital health was. By 2022 it was so ubiquitous that it was hard to identify anything new or emerging in healthcare delivery that didn't include a "digital health" component.

> In just a few short years, almost no aspect of healthcare will be possible without digital technology.

Sean was the first person to open my eyes to how digital was transforming the landscape of healthcare. He compared it with the introduction of ether, which had transformed the field of surgery back in 1846. Prior to that, patients could not be anesthetized, so surgical procedures had to be performed quickly as patients were physically restrained. Surgical technique was limited, and mortality was high, not to mention the tremendous pain and suffering that was an integral part of any surgical procedure. The advent of ether and more advanced anesthesia created an opening for the types of lengthy, complex, safe, and lifesaving surgical procedures that exist today. Today we don't talk about "ether healthcare" because anesthesia is an integral part of healthcare delivery. There is no such thing as nonanesthesia healthcare. I believe that this will be even more true for digital in that there will be no such thing as nondigital healthcare.

Digital technology already has and will continue to unleash, enable, and amplify the value proposition and immense potential currently locked up in our healthcare delivery system. Its impact will be far greater than any other technological advance to date because it is a networked phenomenon that exists in a continuous, analytically enabled, and autonomous environment. It touches *everyone* in the healthcare universe all the time. Unlike anesthesia, it isn't limited to the surgical suite or one aspect of healthcare delivery, and it is far more fluid and connected than any medication or device.

To illustrate this point, let's walk through how digitization is transforming the process of a standard doctor's visit.

THE DIGITAL FRONT DOOR OF HEALTHCARE

In the digital health era, instead of knocking on doors or calling receptionists, we'll be entering through the convenience of "the digital front door," where inquiries, scheduling, symptom checking, referrals, and preference routing can be automated through an app or website set up by your provider network. The ideal digital front door will offer numerous services, including the following:

The ability to go online and find the right provider for you. Through the health system's portal, you'll be able to match with the professional you want to entrust with your health. Maybe you want an older provider with years of experience, or perhaps the gender of the doctor is important to you. Or maybe you want a provider who is race concordant or one who shares a similar cultural background. This advanced matching technology already exists, and it's just a matter of time before it becomes a fixture in the digital health foyer.

Online appointment scheduling. At this point in time, online scheduling is pretty much commonplace in most large delivery networks. You can schedule appointments prioritized by a convenient location and drive time, by availability, or by the type of provider you're looking for.

Automated triage. Automated and semiautomated "symptom checkers" are commonly used by healthcare systems, provider groups, and freestanding urgent care centers and emergency departments. This empowers patients to have a sense of the acuity and severity of their symptoms; in a sense, automated triage is a self-triage tool.

"E-visits." A variant of the symptom checker is what some refer to as an "e-visit." There is an automated, branched-logic series of questions you fill out and respond to online. The results of this online questionnaire are packaged, prepped, and sent to your provider, who will email you back within a few hours. E-visits go beyond triage to actual diagnosis and treatment. The key is that it's asynchronous, meaning that you and the provider don't have to be in the same place or communicating at the same time.

"Virtual visits." This is a synchronous visit where both you and the provider are communicating at the same time either by telephone (voice only) or with video enhancement. These types of visits are now fairly commonplace and are offered by providers and hospital systems as well as by insurance companies, with the tech and platform often supplied by telehealth companies. The providers conducting virtual visits can be aided by a software symptom checker or by an evidence-based, up-to-date symptom algorithm. The point is to rapidly and conveniently establish the level of urgency, obtain a diagnosis, order supportive lab tests or imaging studies, provide immediate treatment, and refer to another setting, such as an emergency room, an urgent care, a primary care, or a specialist.

All of these digitized visits can be offered not just for clinical problems but also for administrative purposes—addressing issues such as payment, insurance coverage and benefits, scheduling, referrals, and prior authorizations needed for tests or referrals.

Utilizing the digital front door means a lot of time-saving prep will happen before you step into the provider's office. These interactions are rapidly becoming a reality, thanks to entrepreneurs such as Brandon Robertson, whose company, UCP Merchant Medicine, develops and integrates tools for a comprehensive previsit journey. Here's an example of a patient's journey through the online navigator system, IntelliVisit, that Brandon shared with me:

John is a typical thirty-two-year-old male with no medical conditions who is feeling ill. He's having abdominal pain and nausea. He logs onto a local urgent care website to make an appointment and is connected to a navigator tool. The completely automated navigator allows him the option of an online evaluation to determine whether he should have a virtual visit or an in-person urgent care or primary care visit or head to a local emergency department.

He decides to proceed with the online evaluation, which begins with him entering basic information, such as his name, gender, date of birth, email address, and phone number. After that, the navigator launches into a series of clinically relevant questions and uncovers the medically relevant facts about John's state of health.

John's belly pain, which began the day before, is moderately severe at a six out of ten intensity level. It's located in the left upper quadrant of his abdomen. He's experiencing moderately severe nausea, which began two days ago, but no vomiting, diarrhea, constipation, or discoloration of his stool or urine. There is no chest pain, back pain, or radiation of the pain anywhere else, including his groin, flank, or back. He hasn't traveled anywhere in the past few weeks, no one else in his family is sick, and he hasn't eaten anywhere out of the ordinary. He has three or four glasses of wine per week and does not smoke. There is no history of any drug use. He noticed his recent symptoms while at work eating lunch. Tylenol only helps the pain a little; any activity seems to make the pain worse. He has never had any abdominal conditions or abdominal surgeries in the past and has no past medical history of ulcers, intestinal bleeding, esophagitis, gall-bladder issues, hepatitis, appendicitis, inflammatory or irritable bowel disorders, or kidney stones.

The automated navigator continues to "ask" John questions to further define and refine his symptoms. Once all the questions have been answered, the navigator processes the information and recommends that John seek care at an urgent care center immediately. It attaches a link to schedule an appointment based on the locations and waiting times of nearby facilities. There is also a link to Uber Health, so John doesn't have to worry about transportation.

John arrives at the urgent care via Uber, and the medical assistant (MA) locates his evaluation and confirms his identity. This is where the real magic starts. The automated navigator has already generated a medical encounter and note that includes the symptoms with the most likely diagnoses, what is termed "common considerations." It also recommends a number of specific diagnostics such as blood tests and imaging studies. The MA checks John's vital signs and then carries out the tests recommended by the navigator. In the meantime, an urgent care provider has reviewed the automatically generated chart and is fully aware of the history, assessment, and recommendations produced by the navigator. Once the test results are back, the provider joins John in the exam room, and what might have been a twenty-minute visit literally takes less than five minutes because of all the previsit work. Keep in mind that the time saved can be used to enhance the visit between John and his provider by allowing for more discussion about preventive care and John's lifestyle. In this case, the conclusion is that John has a benign upset stomach. John is given aftercare instructions on what to do if the symptoms don't improve. He's had a frictionless, expedited, and more personalized experience getting the care he needed.

Based on John's example alone, it is clear how this technology can greatly elevate the patient experience. If you're thinking, "I'd rather talk to a person, not a computer," then you would be missing out on some huge advantages of this kind of system. These include the following:

24/7 access. If you have a concern in the middle of the night, you no longer have to wait until morning to get guidance. You can find out at that moment if your condition is serious enough to seek immediate care.

Speed of response. The digital front door will automatically connect you with the right resources in your healthcare system. Keep in mind that the software and analytics can instantly access not only your medical records but also your healthcare insurance and financial information, as well as the schedules and availability of all the providers and resources in the health system. There are no long delays, no looking up information, no callbacks, and no waiting. Instead, the information is stored, analyzed, updated, and delivered back to you instantaneously, thanks to AI, which has the capacity to quickly provide sophisticated and relevant responses. (We'll return to AI in a moment and do a deeper dive throughout the chapter.)

Reduction in human resources and cost. This technology does not negate the need or disrupt the desire to interact with a healthcare provider. The optimal situation could be a hybrid offering, not only empowering you with this incredible technology but also affording you the opportunity to interact with a person either synchronously or asynchronously. Utilizing this approach, we can greatly reduce the number of resources required by having the digital responses up front. This will also reduce the costs of care while improving the experience and outcomes.

Democratization of data. In the old days (like twenty years ago), most healthcare documentation was handwritten. You would enter a doctor's office and see piles of paper charts strewn about. What you may have not noticed was something we used to call a "file room," where all the paper charts were stored. (Hospitals had entire floors filled with paper charts.) If that doctor, an assistant, or a nurse accidentally wrote something down incorrectly, forgot to note something important, or misfiled your information, good luck. In contrast, through digital technology, your healthcare information will be retained, sorted, and easily shared with whatever professionals provide your care. It can also be analyzed by sophisticated quality and safety software to catch errors, flag discrepancies and other issues, and improve the health of populations. Importantly, all that information will be available to you as well.

One last point to note here. While we've focused here on the previsit, all of this will be utilized in the postvisit and between-visit time as well.

HOW DIGITAL HEALTH AND AI ARE REHUMANIZING HEALTHCARE

It's important to acknowledge that John's scenario might raise some concerns. Folks may start to believe their care is in the hands of computers, not people. That's simply not the case. The final responsibility and decision-making for your actual treatment still rests squarely on the providers' shoulders, not with the chatbot. The online portal is gathering the time-consuming information that providers and other medical workers would have had to pause to write down and file. Your providers save valuable time, and you're saved from filling out form after form. And one really important aspect of all this—*your doctor now has more time to attend to you.* Thanks to this automated prep, you can receive greater attention and more personalized care. Advances in AI will continue this positive trend.

I'd like to introduce you to Dr. Eric Topol, if you aren't already aware of who he is—an internationally renowned cardiologist and researcher, the founder and director of the Scripps Research Translational Institute, and one of the top ten most cited medical researchers in the world. Dr. Topol has been voted the #1 most influential physician leader in the United States by *Modern Healthcare*. He's also one of the most outspoken physicians on the issue of patient advocacy and, in his own words, "patient activism." Eric firmly believes that the use of AI in medical practice will improve diagnostic accuracy, reduce medical errors, lower healthcare costs, enhance providers' productivity, and greatly leverage providers' time, leading to significant increases in access. But even more than that, he believes that AI will actually restore the "human factor" that has been lost in the practice of medicine. This is a premise he discusses in detail in his best-selling book *Deep Medicine: How Artificial Intelligence Can Make Healthcare Human Again*. To Topol, AI will empower providers by freeing up enough of their time and attention to instead focus on being empathetic experts, guides, and teachers to their patients. As Eric explained in a podcast interview I conducted with him, his concern is that personalized, relationship-centered care will continue to deteriorate unless we more readily adopt and integrate AI into daily medical practice.

WHAT ABOUT THOSE WHO AREN'T COMFORTABLE WITH TECHNOLOGY?

Another concern about automated response systems or chatbots is that older patients and some others won't feel comfortable using them or that automated systems might not be sophisticated enough to deal with the more complex conditions that seniors encounter. Meet Alex Harb. Alex is the founder and CEO at Lena Health. Lena Health is a call center service for seniors that utilizes a hybrid approach: chatbot responses, SMS text messaging, and phone calls with lay health navigators. Alex had previously worked within the internationally renowned Texas Medical Center (TMC) to research and understand how they provide support to their senior patients. He analyzed thousands of lines of transcripts from nursing and care coordinator call centers across the multiple healthcare systems within TMC. What he discovered was that 92 percent of the call requests from seniors were questions that were logistical or administrative in nature, not clinical. In other words, nurses didn't need to triage a symptom or provide direct clinical support but were instead guiding patients on issues such as scheduling an appointment or making a referral. Surprisingly, a lot of these questions came in the form of "My doctor told me that I need to go see a cardiologist, and he told me the name, but I got home, and I forgot. Can you tell me which cardiologist I should go see?"

Alex described this discovery as a "light bulb moment." He initially believed that most of the questions seniors called in with were about clinical or complex psychosocial issues, but the data revealed that the vast majority of the requests made by seniors were unrelated to either clinical needs or psychosocial issues. Instead, they were transactional, task-oriented needs around navigating the healthcare system. Furthermore, he discovered that 80 to 90 percent of these logistical needs could be fully resolved through an automated chatbot without ever needing the intervention of a human navigator. Alex discovered that seniors were incredibly comfortable with the ease and convenience of live chat via SMS texting. In contrast, the literature demonstrates that only 17 percent of adults use electronic medical record portals or download self-service-type apps.[11] So his findings actually pose a solution to one of the industry's long-standing challenges in scaling care coordination and support for the elderly.

---

11   A. Griffin, A. Skinner, J. Thornhill, and M. Weinberger, "Patient Portals: Who Uses Them? What Features Do They Use? And Do They Reduce Hospital Readmissions?" *Applied Clinical Informatics* 7, no. 2 (June 2016): 489–501, https://doi.org/10.4338/ACI-2016-01-RA-0003.

Alex believes that the industry-leading engagement he's achieved is a result of Lena's highly responsive and easy interaction for seniors. But there's another aspect to Lena's success. Lena partners and integrates its own capabilities with those of healthcare practices and large systems. Through these partnerships, Lena is able to automate the majority of patient interactions and escalate calls to its lay health navigators only 10 to 20 percent of the time. The value to healthcare systems, and their senior patients, is profound. Lena's tech-enabled approach allows care coordination teams to scale navigation to many more seniors who previously did not have access to navigation assistance.

What's important to recognize here is that human resources in healthcare are limited, and that limitation is beginning to reach crisis level. The nursing and physician shortage may already be noticeable to you, and it's getting worse. According to the Bureau of Labor Statistics, the United States is facing a nursing shortage of over 200,000 nurses each year that is projected to continue throughout the next decade, largely due to the combination of increased demand and nursing retirements.[12] The physician issue is also dire, with an estimated shortage of between 37,800 and 124,000 physicians by 2034.[13] Aside from the costly long-term solution of training up more providers, digital technologies will enable fewer providers to provide care to many more patients. If we can reduce the number of nurses required to manage a call center, as Lena is doing, that helps create capacity for when a nurse is actually needed.

And then there's the cost issue. Each additional nurse added to a call center is at least $100,000 per year in expense, with a maximum

---

12   "Nursing Shortage," American Association of Colleges of Nursing, October 2022, https://www.aacnnursing.org/news-information/fact-sheets/nursing-shortage.

13   "AAMC Report Reinforces Mounting Physician Shortage," Association of American Medical Colleges, June 11, 2021, https://www.aamc.org/news-insights/press-releases/aamc-report-reinforces-mounting-physician-shortage.

capacity of 300 patients. Some early results verify the cost savings Lena has created. Houston Methodist Coordinated Care (HMCC) is an Accountable Care Organization that has partnered with Lena to care for frail elderly patients with complex conditions. HMCC partnered Lena Health with their own nurse navigator program. In a 2021 retrospective claims study, they observed significant reductions in avoidable ED visits, hospitalizations, and readmissions. That led to a 29 percent decrease in total costs of care, translating into annual savings of $3,279 per patient. Patient engagement metrics were equally impressive, with 87 percent enrollment success, 88 percent active monthly usage by patients, and a net promoter score (NPS) of 92.[14] For those unfamiliar with NPS, it's a commonly used industry metric that measures consumers' satisfaction with their experience. A score of 60 or 70 places you in the solid realm of an Apple-like consumer experience. A score in the 90s is stellar.

Although Alex's focus is on the transactional care coordination and navigation needs of older patients, and while the product is highly tech-enabled through the use of AI, it's clear that Lena's fundamental purpose is to humanize healthcare. As Alex states, "For me, it's about how do we improve the aging experience of our seniors and how do we build solutions that are based on human touch and connection that can be maintained throughout their experience."

THE APPOINTMENT

In the patient example we described earlier, all that was required for John was a relatively straightforward visit to an urgent care center. That clearly will not be the case for all patients. So how does the digital

---

14   "Concierge Health Assistant Reduced Costs of Care by 29% Representing $3,279 in Savings per Patient Annually: Retrospective Claims Study," Lena Health, 2021, www. lena.io.

transformation play out once you're inside the provider's office or inside the walls of the hospital? The advantages of the previsit hold true here as well. One study from the University of Minnesota School of Public Health found that primary care providers (PCPs) spend an average of 18 minutes with each patient.[15] A related study from Cerner, the electronic health record vendor, examined 100 million patient visits across 155,000 doctors of all specialties and found that providers spend 16.25 of those 18 minutes using the electronic health record (EHR), most of that while in the room with the patient. PCPs had even higher EHR usage, in the range of 18–22 minutes per patient.[16] Simple math tells us that doctors, on average, are spending less than 5 minutes per visit actually examining and delivering direct care to patients. That's a grossly suboptimal amount of time, hardly enough for a value-laden experience, for either patient or doctor. In emerging models of healthcare, and as a result of digital enablement, providers will have more time to establish a meaningful and trusting relationship with their patients, fully answer questions, address concerns, and provide more personalized guidance and treatment.

Here's what's coming: As your provider is examining you, there will be a software program running in the background that will help guide them in making clinical decisions about your overall health. We call software programs such as

> As a result of digital enablement, providers will have more time to establish a meaningful and trusting relationship with their patients.

---

15 Hannah T. Neprash et al., "Measuring Primary Care Exam Length Using Electronic Health Record Data, *Medical Care* 59, no. 1 (January 2021): 62–66, https://doi.org/10.1097/MLR.0000000000001450.

16 Marc Overhage and David McCallie Jr., "Physician Time Spent Using the Electronic Health Record during Outpatient Encounters: A Descriptive Study," *Annals of Internal Medicine* 172, no. 3 (February 4, 2020): 169–174, https://doi.org/10.7326/M18-3684.

these "decision support tools"—sophisticated digital programs that are triggered whenever your doctor orders a medication or a test. Scott Weingarten, a physician executive and serial entrepreneur, describes how this works.

> *You have lower back pain, and your doctor has just ordered an MRI of your lower back. "Hearing" this, the software will kick in and inform your physician, instantaneously, that this test is not recommended by widely accepted evidence-based guidelines. Conversely, if the software senses another test is needed, it will remind the doctor to order it, based on the diagnosis. A lot of the software programs that are running right now are far from perfect. But they're getting better—far more efficient and focused. In fact, they're actually reducing the number of less valuable alerts that physicians and other providers are receiving—both in the offices as well as in hospitals.*

This type of software will be at work even when you're *not* seeing the doctor, in what might be called the "between visit" phase, which is where we spend most of our lives. At this point in time, many healthcare systems have software programs running all the time, analyzing your information, and looking for opportunities to be much more proactive and preventive both in the hospital and outside of it. One wonderful example of this is algorithms that look for missing preventive screening tests, such as mammograms or colonoscopies, that can identify cancers early before they require surgery or chemotherapy or before they're untreatable.

These digital software programs scan your medical records looking for "care gaps"—some test or other element of care that you're due, or overdue, for. When they come across one, they will alert your doctor or healthcare system that you need to be called to come in. Some of these programs will also send automatic alerts directly to you. Why shouldn't this be the case? After all, your smartphone is "thoughtful" enough to remind you when to install an operating system update. Isn't your health important enough to warrant those types of alerts?

The digital world offers you, as a patient and consumer, far more agency over your own healthcare because now you don't have to wait for a visit with your physician, and you don't have to wait for alerts. In many healthcare systems today, you can go online and check for yourself if you're due for any preventive screenings or treatments.

Now let's return to your in-person visit and look at one more piece of technology that is changing things up in a tangible and important way. When a physician examines you, you probably notice that they're recording their findings, including your medical history, the physical examination, and any diagnoses, as well as creating a problem list and plan of action. At the present time, most providers are still physically typing this information into the electronic health records database. Some providers are dictating it, either during or after the visit. But coming soon, the software will be "listening in" on your visit and will be recording the information in real time, including *your perspectives and opinions* as the patient. Not only that, but the software will also provide immediate feedback on the diagnostic possibilities and likelihoods, as well as advising on recommended tests and treatments. The digital analytics will literally "feel" like a real-time expert consultant in the room. Again, it won't replace, minimize, or detract from the human-to-human interaction. Quite the opposite could occur because your provider will be freed from having to record and look up information. That energy, time, and attention can be redirected to focusing on you as a person. If the doctor misunderstands something you've said, you can more easily correct it, in real time, as it's being automatically recorded and shared with both of you. You can also insert your preferences, which are always important in clinical decision-making but often overlooked. These examples are what Dr. Topol was referring to when he so brilliantly articulated that far from dehumanizing the healthcare experience, digital enhancement will rehumanize it.

What's astounding to me, and might be to you as well, is that these technological capabilities already exist. For example, Cerner is working with Amazon's Transcribe Medical to develop a "digital voice scribe" that will translate the patient-doctor conversation into the appropriate fields in the EHR.[17] Google has recently launched its own AI-enabled conversational product, dubbed "Bard." Microsoft purchased Nuance for $16 billion in 2022 and has codeveloped a conversational AI platform.[18] Nuance's tool, Dragon Ambient eXperience (DAX) Express, utilizes the next iteration of AI language software, ChatGPT-4, which will be available in private preview the summer of 2023. As Mark Benjamin, CEO of Nuance, stated, "We are marking the next step forward in the ongoing evolution of AI-powered solutions for overburdened care providers."[19] And there are many more companies generating these sophisticated services. The technology is here; it's just not yet everywhere. But it soon will be, for just about every type of medical, surgical, or behavioral specialty encounter.

---

17   Lily Lieberman, "Cerner Exec: 'Grand Vision' for Digital Voice Scribe Is to Eliminate Data Entry for Doctors," *Kansas City Business Journal*, December 9, 2019, https://www.bizjournals.com/kansascity/news/2019/12/09/cerner-amazon-aws-digital-voice-scribe.html.

18   "Microsoft Completes Acquisition of Nuance, Ushering in New Era of Outcomes-Based AI," Microsoft News Center, March 4, 2022, https://news.microsoft.com/2022/03/04/microsoft-completes-acquisition-of-nuance-ushering-in-new-era-of-outcomes-based-ai/.

19   Emily Olsen, "Microsoft's Nuance Reveals Clinician Note-Taking Tool with GPT-4," *MobiHealthNews*, March 21, 2023, https://www.mobihealthnews.com/news/microsofts-nuance-reveals-clinician-note-taking-tool-gpt-4?.

THE DIGITAL DIVIDE

Another concern is that digital technology will worsen the growing disparities and inequities in healthcare, whether that be along racial lines, or tied to poverty, or in rural environments. Thankfully, what we're actually seeing is the beginning of the "democratization" of healthcare delivery. By democratization, we mean making care more accessible, more affordable, more convenient, and more customizable to a much wider audience and thereby crossing the so-called "digital divide" to provide care to underserved segments of the American public. The evidence for this crossing of the digital divide is mounting. As healthcare moves into the home and to the point of need (which we'll learn more about in chapters 2 and 3), systems are using portable Wi-Fi hubs to establish internet and Bluetooth connectivity. And at this very moment in time, the federal government is deploying a $50 billion bipartisan initiative to bring high-speed internet networks to households across the country. This initiative, which should be completed this decade, coupled with the increasingly sophisticated, lower cost, and more ubiquitous digital technologies, will address the social determinants of health (SDOH) and serve to decrease healthcare disparities and inequities. It will enable underserved individuals, families, and communities by giving them greater options, more autonomy, and more control over their healthcare and their health.[20] In fact, according to government officials I've spoken to, access to telehealth is one of the top priorities that families specify when asked about the importance of high-speed internet placement in their homes.

---

20 "Advancing Racial Equity and Support for Underserved Communities through the Federal Government," US Department of Commerce Equity Action Plan, January 20, 2021, https://www.commerce.gov/sites/default/files/2022-04/DOC-Equity-Action-Plan.pdf.

THE TIP OF THE ICEBERG

This chapter covered the proverbial tip of the iceberg by providing a very quick glimpse into the vast terrain of the digitization of healthcare. We've only scratched the surface of what is available and emerging. At this point in time, there are over 2,500 digital healthcare companies in existence.[21] In addition, a 2021 IQVIA Institute for Human Data Science Trends report described that more than 90,000 digital health apps had been released in 2020—an average of two-hundred fifty per day. They also reported that, by 2021, there were already more than 350,000 digital health apps on the market.[22] As someone who has been tracking these advances for years, I'll freely admit that they're being developed and deployed at an accelerated pace that is challenging to keep up with. Below are a few other cutting-edge digital medical services that already exist. These are largely off-the-shelf technologies with the potential to radically improve care, reduce healthcare costs, and democratize care.

1. Software that will alert your healthcare system or provider if you're admitted to a hospital or discharged (e.g., Patient Ping from Bamboo Health)

2. AI-enabled software that can read pathology reports and imaging studies, improving diagnostic accuracy, reducing costs, and scaling care to the underserved both here in the United States and across the globe (e.g., QuantX from Qlarity Imaging, Oncotopix Discovery from Visiopharm)

---

21   "Discover Top Digital Health Startups in United States," Health Tech Alpha, March 25, 2023, https://www.healthtechalpha.com/country/digital-health-startups-in-united-states.

22   Emily Olsten, "Digital Health Apps Balloon to More Than 350,000 Available on the Market, according to IQVIA Report," *MobiHealthNews*, Aug. 4, 2021, https://www.mobihealthnews.com/news/digital-health-apps-balloon-more-350000-available-market-according-iqvia-report.

3. A digital platform that can be used by you or your provider to order any service with a digital footprint (e.g., Xealth from Maven Clinic)

4. A digital platform that will allow patients and providers across multiple hospital systems to consult one another and share data (e.g., Care Everywhere from Epic)

5. Digital apps and platforms that are bringing much-needed behavioral health to children and adults across the nation (e.g., Charlie Health, Cerebral, Ginger, Headspace, Talkspace, MoodKit, I Am Sober, AbleTo, BetterHelp, MindShift, Happify)

There's an important point I made earlier in this chapter that bears repeating. These efforts aren't about replacing the provider-patient relationship; they're about enhancing it. I've interviewed dozens of experts in digital health, and each time I do, they tell me their motivation is to go "back to the future"—to recreate care that is more relational and personalized. My hope is that you view digital tech as an enabler, providing us with easy-to-use tools that reduce the burden on providers, reduce the friction for patients, and create the space for more meaningful and value-laden connections.

But as with everything else in life, there are always unintended consequences. With the introduction of the thousands of digital health companies and applications, there is the serious risk of introducing greater complexity and fragmentation into healthcare. We are already witnessing and experiencing this as the digital health vendors vie for adoption

> These efforts aren't about replacing the provider-patient relationship; they're about enhancing it.

and use within hospital systems, provider groups, payers, and the newer retail entrants. This challenge is not going away, but there are solutions, some of which we'll be discussing later on, that can support healthcare leaders and managers in navigating and curating the new world order of digital health.[23]

HELLO, ChatGPT

In the few months that passed between the original writing of this chapter and its final edit, we witnessed another example of the ferocious acceleration and amplification of the digital revolution. In November 2022 the OpenAI platform ChatGPT was introduced—an advanced generative AI technology that is vastly superior to anything seen before.

In fact, the original version passed the US medical licensing exam.[24] Not surprisingly, there was immediate speculation and concern that it could soon replace the judgment of physicians. Fueling these concerns, the pace of ChatGPT's development has so far been staggering. Within a short time, that original version has been updated to ChatGPT4. If it follows the path of other new technologies, ChatGPT will likely traverse the famed Gartner hype cycle, moving from the "peak of inflated expectations" to the "trough of disillusionment" to the "slope of enlightenment," landing at the "plateau of productivity."[25] We're at the peak right now, and it's been so daunting that it's even put the likes of Elon Musk on the defensive, as he and

---

23   Ann Aerts and Doreen Bogdan-Martin, "Leveraging Data and AI to Deliver on the Promise of Digital Health," *International Journal of Medical Informatics* 150, no. 104456 (June 2021): ISSN 1386–5056, https://doi.org/10.1016/j.ijmedinf.2021.104456.

24   Tiffany H. Kung et al., "Performance of ChatGPT on USMLE: Potential for AI-Assisted Medical Education Using Large Language Models," *PLOS Digital Health* 2, no. 2 (2023): e0000198, https://doi.org/10.1371/journal.pdig.0000198.

25   "Gartner Hype Cycle," Gartner, accessed April 17, 2023, https://www.gartner.com/en/research/methodologies/gartner-hype-cycle.

a few other illuminati have actually petitioned for a moratorium in it and other AI-driven technology's development.[26]

In the medical domain, seminars have been held, articles have been published, and numerous books have already been written about the impact generative AI will have on healthcare delivery.[27] In an interesting twist, physician and Wharton Business School professor David Asch actually interviewed ChatGPT on its potential to improve healthcare. In this interview, Dr. Asch and ChatGPT "discussed" issues such as opportunities and benefits, challenges in adoption and integration, and the concerns and fears that have been raised by physicians. They also addressed tough-to-solve issues such as healthcare inequities, the mental health crisis, and the alleviation of clinician burnout.

Here are a few of ChatGPT's responses to the question, "What are the big opportunities for using ChatGPT in healthcare?"

1. Virtual assistants for patient care: ChatGPT could be used to create virtual assistants who can help patients schedule appointments, answer medical questions, and provide information on symptoms and treatments.

2. Clinical documentation: ChatGPT could be used to automate the process of creating clinical documentation, such as medical charts and progress notes.

3. Medical research: ChatGPT could be used to analyze large volumes of medical data and assist in the discovery of new treatments and cures.

---

26 Matt O'Brien, "Musk, Scientists Call for Halt to AI Race Sparked by ChatGPT," Associated Press, March 29, 2023, https://apnews.com/article/artificial-intelligence-chatgpt-risks-petition-elon-musk-steve-wozniak-534f0298d6304687ed080a51 19a69962.

27 Peter Lee, Carey Goldberg, and Isaac Kohane, *The AI Revolution in Medicine: GPT-4 and Beyond* (London: Pearson, 2023); Harvey Castro, *ChatGPT and Healthcare: The Key To New Future of Medicine*, independently published, 2023.

4. Medical education: ChatGPT could be used to create interactive educational tools for medical students.

5. Patient engagement: ChatGPT could be used to create chatbot-based applications for patient engagement, providing patients with real-time feedback and support for self-management of their care.

ChatGPT also commented on its own limitations: "One of the biggest concerns when using ChatGPT in healthcare is the potential for data breaches and unauthorized access to sensitive patient information" and its potential biases. "ChatGPT is trained on large amounts of data, which may contain biases. This can lead to the model making biased predictions, which can have a negative impact on patient care. It is important to ensure that the data used to train the model is diverse and representative of the population it will serve."

Toward the end of the interview, Dr. Asch asked ChatGPT to write a poem based on their conversation. Here is what ChatGPT came up with:

This interview has been quite a ride,
With questions on healthcare to guide,
ChatGPT's capabilities we explored,
And many insights were outpoured.
From financial risks to patient care,
We delved deep into what's fair.
With technology's role in mind,
We hope to leave the future kind.[28]

---

28 David Asch, "An Interview with ChatGPT about Healthcare," *NEJM Catalyst*, April 4, 2023, https://catalyst.nejm.org/doi/full/10.1056/CAT.23.0043.

I found those last couple of lines particularly relevant to one of our central themes in this book and somewhat surprising coming from an AI algorithm.

The opportunities and benefits for ChatGPT underscore what we've discussed in this chapter. Some of the challenges to its adoption will be the security and regulatory hurdles and its integration into existing platforms. There is no question that accuracy, safety, and reliability will have to be tested prior to its adoption. It's unclear if the FDA will be regulating ChatGPT, as it's not yet labeled a medical device or treatment. Some regulators are already lobbying for AI software to be treated as a medical device.[29]

There is much speculation about the future role and safety of AI software such as ChatGPT, but there are a few things I feel fairly comfortable saying at this point. First, the sophistication of this technology will continue to advance very quickly. There is more than enough interest from investors as well as from technologists and scientists. Second, healthcare consumers will continue to use the technology as long as it's available. Third, in keeping with the viewpoint I've expressed throughout this chapter, this technology will not eliminate the need for physicians. ChatGPT corroborated this last point eloquently during its interview with Dr. Asch. Per ChatGPT, "It's true that the capabilities of AI and machine learning … are rapidly advancing. However, it's important to remember that [while] ChatGPT … can generate human-like text, it does not have the ability to think, reason, or understand the context of the information it generates…. Human healthcare professionals have a deep understanding of the nuances of healthcare and the emotional and social context of their patients, and this is something that ChatGPT can't replicate."

---

29   Nabil Shaikh, "Is Your Phone a Medical Device?" *The Regulatory Review*, February 28, 2023, https://www.theregreview.org/2023/02/28/shaikh-is-your-phone-a-medical-device/.

In the next chapter, we'll dive into a new ecosystem of care that is being created outside of the concrete walls of the hospital, emergency department, and clinic. Remember when doctors made house calls? Well, you're about to learn how the house call is making a big digitally enabled comeback and is being reframed as a home-based healthcare ecosystem.

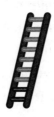

CHAPTER 2

THE POINT OF NEED IS NOW THE POINT OF CARE

The healthcare ecosystem has traditionally been built for the healthcare ecosystem. Instead, let's put the patient at the center.
—Dr. Jennifer Schneider, CEO and cofounder, Homeward

Until relatively recently, if you needed to purchase something, you had to get yourself to a store. Sure, you could mail order from a catalog, but it wasn't all that convenient or common. Today you can order almost anything and have it delivered to your front door within days to even hours—clothes, shoes, groceries, books, pens, toilet paper, you name it. Even meals can be ordered and delivered to your door within minutes.

Until relatively recently, if you wanted to watch a movie, you had to get yourself to a movie theater. Sure, you could watch movies on TV, but it wasn't all that convenient, and the selection was greatly limited. Today you can watch almost anything you want anytime and have it streaming on any screen you own anywhere you are.

Until relatively recently, if you needed medical attention, you had to get yourself to an urgent care center, or your doctor's office, or the emergency department. Today you can receive different levels of medical care—urgent care, emergency room care, primary care, specialty care, and even hospital-level care—all from the comfort, convenience, and safety of your own home.

This advance was greatly catalyzed by the COVID-19 pandemic, but it has been in development for over a decade, thanks to the humanistic vision of numerous entrepreneurs. Sean Duffy, whom you were introduced to in chapter 1, is one of those visionaries who has helped shift the point of care from the healthcare center to the center of your life. Sean was obsessed with two things as a young man: medicine and technology. After spending two years at Google in the early 2000s and soaking up the power of the internet, he decided to simultaneously earn an MD degree at the Harvard School of Medicine and an MBA at the Harvard School of Business. Then in 2010 he had a startling realization and left both schools.

Harvard Medical School is located in Boston's Longwood area, near numerous hospitals and medical centers. Sean came to this area for classes, and he couldn't help but notice the thousands of patients walking or driving or taking public transport, heading to see their physicians. The same question kept popping up in his head: "Why do all these people have to come here? *Why don't we go to them?*"

Asking himself this question altered his career and his life—and it's probably already impacting yours.

SHIFTING TO THE POINT OF NEED

Let's start by considering the title of this chapter, "The Point of Need Is Now the Point of Care." The point of need is where any individual who requires medical treatment happens to be—where they live, where they work, where they socialize. Until recently, "the point of care" has largely referred to a physical location where healthcare is provided by medical professionals—a medical practice or emergency room or a hospital. But thanks to the digital enablement discussed in chapter 1, the system is shifting the point of care to the point of need. As Sean Duffy realized over a decade ago, we need to get beyond the centralized, industry-centric paradigm of care. For those of us who are healthcare professionals, our whole way of working has been based upon the point of care being where *we* are, not where our patients are. It's also based on care being delivered in a single point in time, even though patients' needs don't start and stop during an office visit. This legacy approach made sense, given the available technology at the time. But the limitations of the past can be transcended by the digital tools now at our disposal. Now the point of care can shift to the point of need and away from an episodic office visit to care that is continuously available.

Back to Sean's journey. After he left both graduate schools, he began to study digital enablement. Because of his time at Google, he understood enough to know what was possible. Now he needed to know how to make it a reality. So he spent time at IDEO, a design consultancy dedicated to innovation breakthroughs, and he also wrote for and was an editor at Medgadget, a popular medical technology blog. Finally, in 2011 he made his move. He became cofounder and CEO of Omada Health and began trying out his ideas for digitally delivering tools to help people care for themselves wherever they happened to be.

Sean decided to start with diabetes. He adapted a sixteen-week course, the National Diabetes Prevention Program, in which participants meet once a week to learn about the chronic condition known as prediabetes and how to reduce their risk of transitioning into full-blown diabetes. The content of the course focused on nutrition, physical activity, cooking, and self-care. He took the entirety of the in-person classroom content and converted it into a completely online, digital prediabetes program.

It turns out that the online program is just as good in terms of the medical outcomes achieved, and it's a more personalized experience. You can sign up from the comfort of your own home. You receive a personality assessment designed to customize your experience. The assessment also puts you into a cohort with people who are psychologically compatible and assigns a coach who fits your personality profile. All of this helps create the optimal environment for motivation, accountability, social support, sustained engagement, and behavior change. You attend the sixteen-week educational course, but it's offered asynchronously, so you don't have to be anywhere at any set time. You can log in any time of day or night, view the course material and content, ask your coach questions, and interact with the other participants. You are sent a Bluetooth scale that connects to your smartphone, along with a kit of other helpful tools. Your progress is compared with others in an anonymous way. The result is a cohesive local community that is digitally enabled and designed to motivate much-needed behavior changes. The interactive elements enable users to fully engage with all they need to know about diabetes as well as their own progress in dealing with it.

Not only is this a far superior experience for the patient. It's more effective too. Omada reports that employers and payers save, on average, $1,000 per member in the first year their service is used. Their diabetes program has also shown meaningful reductions in participants' hemoglobin A1C levels and cholesterol levels.[30]

Contrast this with the old-school way of dealing with diabetes—you travel to a doctor's visit, where you receive a brief but dense tutorial on diabetes as well as a generic list of the changes you need to make in your life. How much will you actually remember from that encounter? And how much of that will help you make and maintain the complex and challenging behavior changes needed to achieve success? Probably not a lot.

As Sean shared during one of our podcast interviews, "Getting someone to work on their lifestyle, change behavior, and lose a modest amount of weight requires so many touch points and interactions. And you can get that in person, no doubt.... But the limited frequency with which you get to connect with people in those in-person programs means that it has limited scalability. It felt like digital had to be a solution here. And people are increasingly spending more time in front of their screens, so you have to meet them where they are."

A couple of things fueling this trend of the point of care being delivered at the point of need are not only that it's scalable, but also that it's actually more engaging, more informative, and more useful. Your treatment doesn't end when you leave the office visit. Instead, it's a continuous, 24/7 process designed to keep you as healthy as possible with as little disruption in your daily life as possible. To the point of scalability, I recently spoke with Sean, who shared with me that Omada is now available to one out of every ten commercially insured

---

30 "Evidation Study Validates Key Outcomes for Omada Diabetes Program," Omada, September 2, 2020, https://resourcecenter.omadahealth.com/press-releases/evidation-study-validates-key-outcomes-for-omada-diabetes-program.

adults in the United States as part of their employee health benefits. Underpinning this megatrend is the transition from a supply-side orientation, in which the point of care is based on the convenience and business model of the provider, to a demand-side orientation, in which the point of care is based on the convenience and needs of the consumer.

Historically, the culture of healthcare delivery has been largely built around the industry itself, *not* around the needs of its consumers or patients. Most industries have evolved to being more consumer-centric in the twenty-first century, providing more information, more choices, and more convenience. Healthcare is late to this particular party but is finally beginning to transform so that the patient-as-consumer is more and more the driver of care delivery.

Within healthcare, there has been a good deal of pushback about thinking of patients as "customers" or "consumers"—as if that kind of designation somehow dehumanized people, turning them into dollar signs. I detail the importance of this distinction in my first book, *Reframing Healthcare*, as well as why this designation is actually *more* humane because it puts the onus on the institution of healthcare to provide their constituents with a higher level of service in order to be successful.[31]

We're finally evolving to a new point of care model where people are increasingly being served where they are rather than in a fixed location, at a fixed point in time, where the provider has "set up shop" and when the "open" sign is on. The point of demand is superseding the point of supply. This transition will be more convenient, produce better outcomes, and also lower costs.

---

31 Zeev Neuwirth, *Reframing Healthcare: A Roadmap for Creating Disruptive Change* (Charleston: Advantage Media Group, 2019), 70–71.

Entrepreneurs Empowering the Shift

Glen Tullman is another highly successful healthcare entrepreneur who is leading the charge in this effort. Currently, Glen is the executive chairman and chief executive officer of Transcarent. He is also a cofounder and the previous CEO of Livongo Health. Both of these companies are expressly dedicated to making the point of care the point of need.

Glen is committed to this objective because he's seen the success of this approach in other industries. Those transformations have allowed those industries to offer 24/7 access as well as more choice, more content, more transparency, and more competitive pricing. When I interviewed Glen, he discussed how this digitally enabled shift to serving consumers has transformed four distinct areas of our lives.

CONTENT

To research something, you used to have to go to a library. That library would have to be open, the books you need would have to be available, and ultimately, your resources would be limited to what's in that single building. After all, no library can stock every single book in the universe. Now all the content in the world can be found through Google or other search engines and, most recently, curated through AI-derived software such as ChatGPT.

COMMUNITY

Social media has opened the door for online communication and community in a way that was unimaginable a few short years ago. We use email, text messaging, Twitter, Snapchat, Instagram, TikTok, and YouTube throughout our daily communications. The Pew Research Center reports that 72 percent of all US adults use at least one social media site. For those under fifty, the number jumps to over 80 percent.[32] These social media platforms have even become verbs such as "insta" and "snap." They've also become sources of revenue. We use Zoom, Teams, and Webex for professional and personal meetings. We have online professional forums to hold seminars with panels and Q and A sessions. We use LinkedIn as a professional platform for communication and networking. This revolution in communication seems essential and irreversible.

COMMERCE

Remember the days when to buy something, you had to go to a mall or store and hope that they had the thing you were looking for? Now most retailers are online, and some don't have a brick-and-mortar location at all. You can go on your phone or laptop, search for the item you want, put in your payment and delivery information, make the purchase, and have it delivered right to your front door.

CARE

Of the four Cs, this one is the new kid in town. Entrepreneurs are now constantly devising ways to deliver healthcare to people at the point of need, particularly those with chronic conditions. Consumers are not only able to monitor such important vital signs as blood pressure, pulse rate, and glucose levels but also receive consistent digital coaching on how best to mitigate their disease's negative aspects.

Glen has been motivated, like most of our 'beyond the walls' entrepreneurs, by the knowledge that people are desperate for change in the healthcare arena. In his own words, "After thirty years of promises for a higher-quality, more cost-effective healthcare system, today people will tell you that it is more confusing, more complex, and more costly than ever before."

---

32   "Social Media Fact Sheet," Pew Research Center, April 7, 2021, https://www.pewresearch.org/internet/fact-sheet/social-media/.

Substantial change requires an understanding of the enabling powers Glen mentions, combined with a mindset that is not anchored in the traditional healthcare model. The care of chronic diseases may be the best example of how this shift to point of care has already been realized.

CHRONIC DISEASE MANAGEMENT AT THE POINT OF NEED

Chronic disease management has become one of the most prominent healthcare challenges of our time. Currently, the vast majority of all medical encounters and the majority of all healthcare dollars are spent on the diagnosis, treatment, and management of chronic disease. In fact, 84 percent of all healthcare costs are attributable to treating chronic diseases.[33] For example, according to the CDC, heart disease and stroke cost the United States $216 billion each year in medical costs and $147 billion in lost productivity. Diabetes is estimated at $327 billion between medical costs and productivity losses.[34] In addition, the downstream impact in terms of financial well-being and costs to life is immeasurable. For example, the incidence rates of mental illness are two to three times higher for individuals with a chronic disease.[35]

Despite the staggering costs and suboptimal outcomes, we continue to treat chronic disease within an episodic, reactive, non-customized, and largely ineffectual care model. In part, this is due to

33 Tara O'Neill Hayes and Serena Gillian, "Chronic Disease in the United States: A Worsening Health and Economic Crisis," American Action Forum, September 10, 2020, https://www.americanactionforum.org/research/chronic-disease-in-the-united-states-a-worsening-health-and-economic-crisis/.

34 "Health and Economic Costs of Chronic Diseases," Centers for Disease Control and Prevention, accessed March 23, 2023, https://www.cdc.gov/chronicdisease/about/costs/index.htm.

35 Grace Fernandez, "The Intersection of Mental Health and Chronic Disease," Johns Hopkins Bloomberg School of Public Health, December 16, 2021, https://publichealth.jhu.edu/2021/the-intersection-of-mental-health-and-chronic-disease.

the predominant fee-for-service (FFS) payment structure that disincentivizes value-based clinical care and value-based business models. It's a reflection of a healthcare delivery approach that is outdated and poorly aligned with our individual and public healthcare needs. The potential, however, to prevent or at least mitigate the impact of chronic disease is enormous.

That's where companies such as Livongo come into play. Its name is based on the phrase "live on the go," which is entirely consistent with an emphasis on the point of care being the point of need. When Glen founded Livongo, he thought it was important to have people within the company who understood, firsthand, what it was like to live with diabetes. As such, nearly one-third of Livongo's employees have diabetes. These are the people who would be using the technology they would develop, so it made sense to have them represented in the workforce. And that included their chief medical officer, Jennifer Schneider, who has type 1 diabetes and who has spoken about it publicly for years.

Livongo's Applied Health Signals program uses data-driven, machine-learning algorithms to deliver continuous, real-time, actionable, and personalized clinical insights rather than rely primarily on doctor visits. The goal is a new era of "human-first experience" in which the locus of chronic condition management shifts from the provider's exam room to the healthcare consumer's life.

I recently interviewed Jennifer, who said, "This idea that the doctor or healthcare provider is in charge is really erroneous. It's really the individual person living with that chronic condition.... The healthcare ecosystem has traditionally been built for the healthcare ecosystem. Instead, let's put the person, the consumer, the patient at the center and build an ecosystem that solves their pain points and empowers them to make decisions that will drive healthful outcomes."

Livongo helps patients deal with chronic conditions such as diabetes, high blood pressure, depression, and weight management. They do this through what they call their "AI+AI" approach, which stands for Aggregate, Interpret, Apply, and Iterate. They begin by collecting as complete a picture as they can of the individual with chronic disease—drawing from multiple data sources such as clinical and pharmacy claims data; EHR data; glucometers, blood pressure, and other physiologic devices; and numerous psychographic and social demographic databases.

They aggregate and analyze this data and then determine a way to present personalized information and recommendations to each individual. Their goal is not just to inform but also to engage and positively influence healthful behaviors through sophisticated tech-enabled behavior change methods. The response from the individual is then fed back into the automated machine-learning software that tracks patterns and analyzes each individual's data to continuously advance personalized communication and interaction.

For example, a patient could measure their glucose level with a finger stick, which would immediately shoot the data through Bluetooth technology to an analytics software program. If the level was too high or too low, the program would automatically respond and tell the patient how to handle it. If the data indicated an urgent need, then the program would engage a diabetic educator who would talk the patient through next steps. And if that patient needed a higher level of care, it would connect them with a doctor or nurse—all in real time.

Responses are immediate when necessary (e.g., if a patient has a low blood sugar reading or a worrisome high blood pressure or signs of mounting anxiety or stress). But the responses are also longitudinal in that they focus on long-term outcomes for each individual. Communication is a hybrid of automated responses and human interaction with health coaches and certified health educators. This sort of process reduces the friction of traditional healthcare delivery by minimizing the frustration and complexity of the patient care experience. Just as importantly, patients are in control of their care and don't have to wait for a doctor visit to see what kind of progress they're making.

At the time of this writing, Livongo has over seven hundred thousand users and has published encouraging outcomes. After one year, members of Livongo's diabetes program saw a 21.9 percent decrease in medical spending, including a 10.7 percent reduction in diabetes-based spending and a 24.6 percent reduction in spending on office visits.[36]

Glen's new start-up, Transcarent (the name is meant to indicate "transparency" and "caring") also delivers cutting-edge methods of bringing care to the point of need. Transcarent can grant a patient almost immediate access to a physician as well as access to a health navigator that can assist in selecting the best and most convenient hospital, surgical group, or healthcare system for the specific type of surgical procedure indicated. The aim is to provide convenient medical advice and care 24/7 with more choice and less cost.

There are three attributes Glen believes need to be in place in order to successfully shift the point of care to the point of need: (1) unbiased information, (2) trusted guidance, and (3) actual connection to healthcare via navigation, scheduling, and making arrangements. The fundamental idea, as Glen points out, is "[to] put the consumer in the driver's seat." This is a far cry from the way most patients and their

---

36   Jonah Comstock, "Lilly-Funded Study Shows Livongo Diabetes Program Can Save Employers $20 to $50 per Member per Month," *MobiHealthNews*, May 9, 2019, https://www.mobihealthnews.com/content/north-america/lilly-funded-study-shows-livongo-diabetes-program-can-save-employers-20-50.

families experience healthcare delivery. As you can see, that negative experience is finally changing for the better.

TELEHEALTH AND A NEW ERA

Telehealth, the ability to have a consultation with a doctor or other medical professional over your phone, tablet, or any internet-enabled device, is another huge aspect of delivering care at the point of need. Its use mushroomed during the pandemic, with telehealth visits in 2020 increasing to 52.7 million from approximately 840,000 in 2019[37] and with 92 percent of these visits occurring in beneficiaries' homes. Telehealth services were critical during the lockdown days when people were unable to go to a doctor's office without risking a COVID-19 infection.

> The fundamental idea is "[to] put the consumer in the driver's seat."

But telehealth had been around for some time before the pandemic made it a necessity. Dr. Roy Schoenberg is another 'beyond the walls' trailblazer and one of the most accomplished entrepreneurs in telehealth and virtual care. He's been at it for over twenty-five years. As the CEO and founder of Amwell, he's built one of the largest telehealth ecosystems in the world.

Roy is also committed to breaking free of the legacy construct of a "visit." He believes there will be three interwoven domains of care delivery in the future.

1. The **physical** care cluster of services in hospitals, operating rooms, clinics, and the like. This is the type of care that was the traditional "go-to."

---

37   Melissa Suran, "Increased Use of Medicare Telehealth during the Pandemic," *JAMA Network Open* 327, no. 4 (January 25, 2022): 313, https://doi.org/10.1001/jama.2021.23332.

2. The **digital (or virtual)** care cluster of services, including telehealth, messaging, and asynchronous communications.

3. **Automated interactions**, which will track, analyze, and engage with patients throughout the course of their healthcare journeys.

Roy believes that once the digital and automated domains are more widely available, care will be much more proactive, personalized, and contextual. For example, automated interactions will end up using tech that has capabilities that our brains simply do not. But we shouldn't look at these new technologies as just add-ons to existing healthcare. In Roy's words, "The part that has changed is that we are beginning to look at telehealth and related technologies more as a logistical infrastructure."

The picture that Roy paints is incredibly positive, hopeful, and attainable. Virtual and digital technologies have the ability to expand access to care to the providers patients want, when patients want it, and how patients want it. From the provider side, those technologies will liberate the tremendous value currently locked up in the hearts and minds of clinicians.

Technology will liberate the tremendous value currently locked up in the hearts and minds of clinicians.

Imagine a healthcare world where clinicians can offer their services not only to the patients within their immediate geography, health system, or network but also to *all* patients, across the country and around the globe. From the public health and industry perspective, digital health will lead to greater efficiencies and effectiveness at far lower costs and will allow us to leverage providers' time much more efficiently, creating unimaginable advances in capacity and population health management.

Most importantly, these new systems are being built around the patients' needs, not the providers'. Let's let Roy have the final word on this amazing revolution:

> *Let's not forget that we are a service industry. We have to que into peoples' lives, not the other way around. Healthcare is just beginning to go through what other industries had gone through ten or fifteen years ago, and the industry has become very hungry for reinventing itself through technology. It will happen much faster than any other revolution healthcare has gone through. This one is for the people, and that is why healthcare is going to change faster than we think.*

In the next chapter, you'll discover a natural progression of this movement—the creation of a home-based care ecosystem—in which your home can be converted into a clinic, an urgent care center, an emergency department, and even a hospital room.

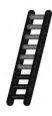

CHAPTER 3

THE HOSPITAL COMES HOME

*The best doctors want to spend time with their patients,
and where better to do that than in the patient's home.*
–Renee Dua, MD, cofounder and CEO, Renee

I n chapter 1 we reviewed how advancements in digital technology have empowered interactions between providers and patients, greatly improving the effectiveness and efficiency of medical care. In chapter 2 we expanded this purview and witnessed how digital enablement is shifting the point of medical care beyond the walls of the healthcare system to where people actually live. We also described the shift from an episodic care system to one that is more continuously responsive to the context of people's lives, improving the experience and care of those with chronic medical conditions as well as those with urgent situations.

This third chapter brings us to a natural continuation of the literal transcendence of the traditional walls of healthcare delivery—where the patient's home can function as a hospital room. As with many of the healthcare disruptions we've discussed, this possibility may seem difficult to believe, but healthcare leaders are doubling down on this breakthrough idea. For example, Roy Jakobs, chief business leader of Connected Care at Philips, has predicted that over the next three years, 40 percent of providers will shift 20 percent of their hospital beds to the home.[38] As Jakobs says, "We can't just serve patients in hospitals. Virtual visits and remote monitoring are going into the home."

That's an idea that one of the most respected consultancy organizations, McKinsey & Company, wholeheartedly agrees with because they believe the hospital-to-home movement will deliver a higher quality of care at a lower price point. Incredibly, they predict up to $265 billion worth of Medicare services (representing up to 25 percent of all Medicare payments) could shift to the home by 2025.[39]

How could this kind of massive change occur in the next couple of years? The answer is that much of it *has already happened*—with the COVID-19 pandemic accelerating the process and forcing many providers to ramp up their virtual visits and home-based care efforts. McKinsey sees four large trends as fueling this hospital-at-home revolution.

Explosive growth in virtual care. Prior to the pandemic, only 11 percent of consumers used telehealth services. By February 2021 the use of telehealth had grown thirty-eight times higher than pre-pandemic levels. Moreover, roughly 40 percent of surveyed consumers said that they expected to continue using telehealth going forward.

More options for post-acute and long-term care needs. Among the increase in the number of elderly patients, the decrease in nursing

---

38   Susan Morse, "The Biggest Trends in Healthcare Are Hospital Care at Home and the Widening Labor Gap," *Healthcare Finance News*, March 22, 2022, https://www.healthcarefinancenews.com/news/biggest-trends-healthcare-are-hospital-care-home-and-widening-labor-gap.

39   Oleg Bestsennyy et al., "From Facility to Home: How Healthcare Could Shift by 2025," McKinsey, February 1, 2022.

home beds (partially a result of the pandemic), the poor quality of many nursing homes, and the psychological impact of the pandemic, a growing number of patients and families are much more open to and even prefer other options for postacute (posthospital) and long-term care, especially now that a combination of remote monitoring, tele-health, social supports, and home modification may enable more patients to receive some level of care at home. According to a survey by AARP, 90 percent of seniors would prefer to stay in their homes as they age, and 82 percent said they would prefer to stay home even if they needed additional care.[40] The survey results should come as no surprise given that 75 percent of nursing homes are understaffed and present an increased risk for falls and opportunistic infections.[41]

Emergence of new technologies and capabilities. New technologies, such as remote monitoring devices, allow providers to keep close watch on patients at home. Again, the pandemic was an accelerant—the Mayo Clinic used remote patient monitoring for ambulatory man-agement of patients with COVID-19 and found that it was effective, with a 78.9 percent engagement rate.[42]

Growing investment in the digital health market. In 2021 venture funding for digital health companies was a record-breaking $29.1 billion as opposed to $14.9 billion in 2020 and $8.2 billion in 2019.[43] While investments lessened a bit the following year, business

---

40   "10 Reasons Why You Should Keep Your Aging Parents in Their Own Home," All Health Choice, accessed March 23, 2023, https://allhealthchoice. com/10-reasons-why-you-should-keep-your-aging-parents-in-their-own-home/.

41   "State of the Nursing Home Industry: Survey of 759 Nursing Home Providers Show Industry Still Facing
Major Staffing and Economic Crisis," American Health Care Association, June 2022, https://www.ahcancal.org/News-and-Communications/Fact-Sheets/FactSheets/ SNF-Survey-June2022.pdf.

42   Bestsennyy et al., "From Facility to Home."

43   Bestsennyy et al., "From Facility to Home."

is backing this movement in a big way, and that means the rapidly emerging digital era will be well financed.

Most thought leaders see the hospital-to-home movement and the shift to a home-based care ecosystem as necessary, inevitable, and imminent. In addition to the trends articulated by McKinsey, here are a couple of other escalating forces. First, the outsize fixed costs of brick-and-mortar hospitals are eroding already thin margins. Second, the increasing costs of supplies and labor are further eroding margins. Since 2019 hospital operating costs have increased by 20 percent, with labor costs up 24 percent and supply costs up 18 percent.[44] Third, lucrative margin-producing procedures continue to move out of the hospital and into ambulatory settings. Fourth, there are capacity constraints given the dwindling number of available nurses due to nursing shortages and the reluctance to work in increasingly more stressful conditions. The net effect is that more hospitals are operating in the red. According to a fall 2022 report released by the AHA, over 50 percent of hospitals were projected to end 2022 with negative operating margins compared to 36 percent in 2019.[45] Even large, highly reputable systems such as Cleveland Clinic, Kaiser Permanente, and Ascension ended 2022 with negative operating margins.

> Most thought leaders see the hospital-to-home movement and the shift to a home-based care ecosystem as necessary, inevitable, and imminent.

---

44   "National Hospital Flash Report," Kaufmann Hall, January 2023, https://www.kaufmanhall.com/sites/default/files/2023-01/KH_NHFR_2023-01.pdf.

45   "The Current State of Hospital Finances: Fall 2022 Update," Kaufmann Hall, 2022, https://www.aha.org/system/files/media/file/2022/09/The-Current-State-of-Hospital-Finances-Fall-2022-Update-KaufmanHall.pdf.

THE HEALTHCARE EARTHQUAKE

One of the trailblazing entrepreneurs in this rapidly advancing area of innovation is Raphael Rakowski. In 2010, years before most of us ever heard of the hospital-at-home concept, Raphael led a team of engineers and clinicians in the creation of Clinically Home, the first commercially scalable model to enable safe hospitalization at home. Then in 2017 Raphael and his team created a next-gen version of Clinically Home called Medically Home, which partnered with Atrius Health, a large multispecialty medical group in Eastern Massachusetts, to bring the program to market. Medically Home now operates in multiple states. Most recently, the company formed a deep strategic partnership with the Mayo Clinic and Kaiser Permanente.

Raphael has no problem calling things the way he sees them. He's a charismatic leader and has a bit of well-earned swagger. He's had a remarkably accomplished, wide-ranging, and multifaceted career as an engineer and entrepreneur, and he's applied that in a groundbreaking way to healthcare delivery. But this isn't just a professional pursuit. His passion for redesigning healthcare comes from a deeply personal place.

Raphael's professional journey began, as he puts it, as "a product guy, a factory guy, an operations guy." After leaving that phase of his career, an initial foray into employer-sponsored healthcare with a company called Empower Health led to him becoming the president of American Healthways, which at the time was a large diabetes disease management company. He grew that business to over three million patients and, in the process, learned how to keep large populations out of the hospital. He next joined the board of a prestigious academic health system. During his board tenure, Raphael's father, a Nazi Holocaust survivor, was admitted to the flagship hospital within that health system. Raphael shares this part of the journey,

My father unfortunately lost his life from three medical errors while I was watching.... And that's how this idea [of a hospital at home] was born. My career has spanned engineering, manufacturing, entrepreneurial start-ups, healthcare services, and a whole bunch of stuff in between. But it ended up with this personal mission on behalf of the experiences that my father had. In his name and in my mother's, trying to make this idea of providing access to safe care for patients in their home, where I believe they want it the most.

Why is it preferable to bring hospital-level care to the home? Echoing the McKinsey report, Raphael makes a convincing case that it comes down to two huge issues: patient safety and financial viability. As Raphael puts it,

Every year, between fifty thousand to one hundred thousand patients die in hospitals from preventable medical errors. That's a dirty little secret that unfortunately is part of an artifact of the way in which we've designed care delivery to try to achieve efficiency. What I discovered was that 65 percent of the cost of that care in a hospital is brick-and-mortar overhead, and it's that overhead that creates a "tax on the care." And when you're left with only 35 percent for clinicians and medical care, it's inadequate. As a result, you have enormous pressure to discharge the patient as quickly as possible because the hospitals get a fixed price for the care.

One of the more remarkable observations Raphael shared is that hospitals were essentially built on a factory model. Raphael knows a bit about factories, as he's built and launched hundreds of them all over the world. His expert opinion is that the hospital-as-a-factory is a fundamentally flawed concept. The same rules that would apply to making cars or textiles or any other widget more efficiently fall apart when applied to the care of people, especially people who are sick and vulnerable enough to be in an acute care setting. Even our accepted notion of acute care and postacute care makes little sense, as he goes on to explain:

> *A patient's care has to continue until they're clinically stable. You can't just say the patient is okay once they're finished with their hospitalization, and now they will be "discharged" and receive postacute care. There is no such thing as postacute care—that's a word that was invented as an artifact of reimbursement. You're not postacute sick and acute sick. You're sick or you're not sick. And you should be cared for by the same care team until you're not sick anymore. Hospital readmission rates are high, at 15 to 20 percent, because [patients] weren't adequately cared for the first time. It's an absolutely blatant signal that the financial and business model of a hospital doesn't work anymore because of the burden of those fixed costs.*

During my correspondence with Raphael, I asked him if he had a critical piece of advice for hospital executives. His answer? "Prepare for an earthquake." When I asked him what he meant by that, he responded, "Because everything you took for granted is being taken away from you." As I said, Raphael is not shy about sharing what he believes, but he's not alone in his belief that things have to change.

THE TRANSPOSITION TO A HOME-BASED CARE ECOSYSTEM

Why abandon the hospital system in favor of one that provides home-based care? The first reason is financial. Circling back to a stunning factoid Raphael provided—the physical brick-and-mortar hospital facility itself, not accounting for any equipment or personnel, accounts for a significant percentage of the cost of a patient's care. Additionally, it costs between $2 million and over $4 million to build the infrastructure surrounding a single hospital bed. Roughly $800 billion per year is spent building hospitals in this country. These are fixed costs, and they have to be paid whether the beds are filled or empty.

So hospitals, like hotels, strive to keep their rooms and beds filled to capacity. This financial imperative drives up the total costs of care for patients and payers. Keep in mind that hospital-based care is the leading cost in American healthcare, at 31 percent of total healthcare expenditures. If you count all the costs that occur as a result of hospitalizations such as in-hospital physician costs and postacute care costs, the number would be even higher.[46] Another factor is hospital bed stays impact patients' health in negative ways. For instance, research shows you could lose up to 40 percent of muscle strength within the first week of immobilization.[47] Most astounding of all, however, is the statistic Raphael alluded to above, that more than four hundred thousand American deaths are associated with preventable harm done to patients in hospital settings.[48]

Clinical labor shortages are another important factor driving the hospital to home transition. According to the American Nurses Association, in 2022 more registered nursing jobs were open than any other profession. With the aging population, the need for nurses will grow by 9 percent in the next ten years. Meanwhile, US nursing

---

46   "Trends in Health Care Spending," American Medical Association, March 20, 2023, https://www.ama-assn.org/about/research/trends-health-care-spending.

47   Selina M. Parry and Zudin A. Puthucheary, "The Impact of Extended Bed Rest on the Musculoskeletal System in the Critical Care Environment," *Extreme Physiology & Medicine* 4, no. 16 (October 9, 2015), https://doi.org/10.1186/s13728-015-0036-7.

48   John T. James, "A New, Evidence-Based Estimate of Patient Harms Associated with Hospital Care," *Journal of Patient Safety* 9, no. 3 (September 2013): 122–128, https://doi.org/10.1097/PTS.0b013e3182948a69.

schools are forced to turn away qualified applicants because they don't have enough faculty or staff.[49] With fewer nurses available or willing to work in the brick-and-mortar hospital setting, we have another factor fueling the trend to home-based hospital level care. All of that seems reason enough to transition the healthcare ecosystem from these high fixed-cost centralized buildings to the home. This may be why major hospital systems such as the Mayo Clinic, Mass General Brigham, Kaiser Permanente, Cleveland Clinic, and Mount Sinai, along with dozens of others, are investing in it. And it's not just the big names. There are literally hundreds of hospital systems investing in hospital-at-home programs. For example, in Medicare's Acute Hospital Care at Home waiver program, there are 115 systems with 276 hospitals in 37 states participating.[50]

So how do we make the transition a seamless one? To pull it off safely and effectively, Raphael informs us that four pillars must be in place.

FOUR PILLARS OF HOSPITAL AT HOME

- Capability to create a hospital room in the home
- Ability to get services into the home in a reasonable time
- Determining and managing the logistics and supply chain
- Creating a "command center"

---

49 "The Truth about the Nursing Shortage—Causes, Statistics, and Solutions," Avant Healthcare Professionals, April 28, 2022, https://avanthealthcare.com/blog/the-truth-about-the-nursing-shortage-causes-statistics-and-solutions.stml.

50 "Acute Hospital Care at Home Resources," Centers for Medicare & Medicaid Services, last updated March 20, 2023, https://qualitynet.cms.gov/acute-hospital-care-at-home/resources.

Pillar 1 is having the capability to recreate a hospital room in the home. That means you have to have the necessary equipment delivered and set up there, including a monitoring system, a communications system, a hospital bed, intravenous (IV) machines, and the appropriate team of clinicians monitoring that equipment virtually.

Pillar 2 is being able to get the services into the home in a reasonable time frame. According to Raphael, there are eighteen or so health services that are generally provided to patients in hospitals, such as dispensing medications, hanging IVs, drawing blood, and delivering oxygen. You must have qualified people available to provide those services in the home, and you must deliver those services in a timely manner to maintain a high standard of care.

Pillar 3 is determining the logistics and supply chains necessary to transport the needed equipment and healthcare workers to the point of care. Those workers must have what they need to provide the same level of care as a traditional hospital would, and protocols must be developed to make sure they can get the proper tools to do so.

Pillar 4 is creating a "command center." This is slightly misleading because the command center doesn't have to be located in an actual physical structure. It can simply be a network of healthcare professionals who are overseeing the patient's care through communication and monitoring systems placed in the patient's home. Those care providers can conduct that oversight in their own living rooms, their offices, or wherever as long as there is a software platform that connects the logistics, the supply chains, the communications, and the integration with the electronic medical records system. This is where Raphael's broad business experience really comes to bear because he believes most people only focus on the clinical part rather than the complex logistics of making the entire hospital-at-home system work. As he says, "This is my background. I'm a logistics expert. This is what I did my entire career. It's not the technology. The technology is there. It's either off the shelf or you can easily buy it or build it. That's not the issue. It's not the clinical expertise. It's not any of that. The thing that is the biggest challenge is the logistics."

It's taken Raphael twelve years to develop his home care model. He prefers not to call what his company does a "hospital at home" because it's not just limited to acute care. Medically Home, such as DispatchHealth and other emerging home-based care provider organizations, can also provide nursing home care, transitional care, long-term care, and even urgent and emergency room care. The ultimate objective is not forcing a patient, especially one who is weak and infirm, to leave their home for care. When a hospital setup is installed in the home, a patient's "discharge" involves removing some of the high-tech equipment and acute care services that are no longer needed. In fact, the discharge from hospital at home is more of a gradual reduction or dialing down of the care and equipment rather than an abrupt removal of everything all at once. If the hospital-at-home patient relapses, the level of care and the equipment are increased and brought back into the home. The intensity of the home care service is modulated up or down according to the patient's needs.

We are seeing some signs that payers are starting to catch up and reimburse hospital care in the home. Centers for Medicare & Medicaid Services (CMS) currently has a waiver program called Acute Hospital Care at Home that was implemented as part of the public health emergency during the pandemic. It has now been extended through December 2024. In the program 250 hospitals and 100 health systems have been granted a waiver to receive reimbursement for hospital-level care in the home.[51] Private insurers have been lagging CMS in terms of payment for hospital-level care in the home, but often, we see the private sector follows the public sector in health care reform. Overall, the future of payment for hospital at home, as well as payment for the entire home-based care ecosystem, is unclear. But one thing is becoming increasingly clear. This is not an issue that's going to be driven by opinion or policy or ideology. The driving forces here will be financial. The current costs of care are unsustainable, and brick-and-mortar hospital-based care will likely have to be reserved for those patients who can't be cared for in their homes.

THE "DARK SIDE OF THE MOON"

We've spent a bunch of time discussing the serious financial imperatives driving the shift to a hospital-at-home model. But there's another compelling reason for building out the home-based care ecosystem. Back in 2021, as part of an initiative being launched at Atrium Health (now Advocate Health), my colleague, Todd Dunn, and I spent a few months interviewing dozens of primary care doctors, geriatricians, nurses, administrators, patients, and family members about home-based care. We participated in a number of home visits as well. One of the doctors I interviewed used the metaphor of the "dark side of the moon" to depict what happens when a patient is discharged from a facility and returns home. He went on to explain that there is an enormous blind spot in the current health system. Unless you go visit the patient at home, and do so regularly, you don't really know what's going on there. You don't know the context of care, which makes it really difficult to provide the type of care and interventions needed,

---

51   Larry Beresford, "Acute Care in the Home Gets Waiver Extension," Medscape, January 4, 2023, https://www.medscape.com/viewarticle/986491#vp_1.

especially for the elderly and patients with more complex chronic conditions.

What that doctor was referring to are all the aspects of homelife that have an outsize impact on health—if the home is safe or not, if the bedsheets are clean or constantly soiled, if there are loose rugs on the floors that can cause a catastrophic fall, if the fridge and cupboards are filled with healthful foods, if there are dozens of expired bottles of medicine in the bathroom or strewn about the kitchen counter, if the electricity and heating are working, if the doors can easily accommodate a wheelchair, if the shower is safe to use and has been outfitted appropriately, if there's enough family and caregiver support around, if the patient is getting any physical activity, if there is enough mental stimulation and interaction with others. And it's more than just knowing whether these arrangements are all in place. It's about being there to deal with whatever issues arise, including shopping for food; preparing meals; picking up prescription medications; assisting with moving about the apartment; climbing stairs; washing clothes; changing bedsheets; paying of bills and managing finances; answering phone calls; dealing with anxiety, depression, and physical pain; and so many other issues that can and do occur.

When care providers are able to enter the home and provide care there on a regular basis, it's like shining a light on the dark side of the moon—identifying the contextual issues, intervening appropriately, and engaging patients, their families, and caregivers in taking all the steps necessary to optimize health.

I acknowledge that before you get discharged from a hospital, there are case managers, social workers, and care managers who come and ask you and your family members questions to help determine that context of care and attempt to secure resources. But how much more effective would it be if medical personnel are actually in your home seeing the situation for themselves? And even though hospital systems have programs in which nurses, nurse practitioners, paramedics, and even physicians do home visits after hospital discharge, these are intermittent and often don't begin until days after the patient leaves the hospital. Quite simply, it's not the same as creating a home-based care ecosystem.

> When care providers are able to enter the home and provide care there on a regular basis, it's like shining a light on the dark side of the moon.

Hospital at Home: The Future of Care

Let's be clear about something—no one believes that brick-and-mortar hospitals will entirely convert into hospitals at home. But if you talk to the experts, they will tell you that anywhere from 30 to 50 percent of current hospitalizations can shift to the home. And other experts have postulated that our current hospitals will niche into specialty care centers, ICU-level care centers, and centers for complex surgical procedures. And while surgical procedures will not be taking place in the home anytime in the foreseeable future, the more common ones have been moving to ambulatory surgical centers (ASCs). In 2017, 95 percent of knee replacement surgeries occurred in the hospital. By the end of 2021, that number had dropped to 25 percent, with the majority being done in ASCs.[52] Similar trends can be said for other common orthopedic procedures such as hip replacements and spine surgery.

The natural consequence of this shift to hospital at home and ASCs will be a downsizing of brick-and-mortar hospital beds. One

---

52 "The Outmigration of Orthopedic Surgeries," Gist Healthcare, August 12, 2022, https://gisthealthcare.com/the-outmigration-of-orthopedic-surgeries-2/.

benefit, of course, will be the reduction in the total costs of care. For currently existing hospital-at-home models, entrepreneurs and researchers have measured costs being lowered by 25 percent.[53] Safety and quality outcomes are also better. A meta-analysis of nine randomized clinical studies showed a lower risk for readmission by 26 percent as well as a lower risk for long-term care admissions compared with the inpatient group.[54] A study published by *JAMA Internal Medicine* with 507 patients found similar results, as well as shorter lengths of stay (3.2 hospital at home versus 5.5 inpatient) and higher patient satisfaction (68.8 percent rated the hospital-at-home experience highly versus 45.3 percent who rated the inpatient experience highly).[55] Finally, the hospital-at-home approach has also demonstrated lower mortality rates, with one study showing 0.93 percent mortality rates for hospital-at-home patients compared with 3.4 percent for inpatient patients.[56] The reduction in mortality is astounding and should draw the attention of hospital and insurance company executives.

As mentioned above, the home-based care ecosystem is expanding beyond hospital at home and encompassing the entire continuum of care. The home care model is also becoming more and more sophisticated. When I spoke to Mark Prather, the CEO and cofounder of

---

53 Bruce Leff et al., "Hospital at Home: Feasibility and Outcomes of a Program to Provide Hospital-Level Care at Home for Acutely Ill Older Patients," *Annals of Internal Medicine* 143, no. 11 (December 6, 2005): 798–808, https://doi.org/10.7326/0003-4819-143-11-200512060-00008.

54 Genevieve Arsenault-Lapierre, Mary Henein, D. Gaid, M. Le Berre, G. Gore, and I. Vedel, "Hospital-at-Home Interventions vs In-Hospital Stay for Patients with Chronic Disease Who Present to the Emergency Department: A Systematic Review and Meta-Analysis," *JAMA Network Open* 4, no. 6 (2021): e2111568, https://doi.org/10.1001/jamanetworkopen.2021.11568.

55 Alex D. Federman et al., "Association of a Bundled Hospital-at-Home and 30-Day Postacute Transitional Care Program with Clinical Outcomes and Patient Experiences," *JAMA Internal Medicine* 178, no. 8 (2018): 1033–1040, https://doi.org/10.1001/jamainternmed.2018.2562https://www.ncbi.nlm.nih.gov/pmc/articles/PMC6143103/.

56 Lesley Cryer et al., "Costs for 'Hospital at Home' Patients Were 19 Percent Lower, with Equal or Better Outcomes Compared to Similar Inpatients," *Health Affairs* 31, no. 6 (2012): 1237–1243, https://doi.org/10.1377/hlthaff.2011.1132.

the highly regarded DispatchHealth home care company, he related that when they first began their efforts back in 2013, they set up a mini emergency room in the back of a Toyota Prius. Over the years, they've morphed into a state-of-the-art home-based care ecosystem that provides care across the continuum—from urgent and emergency care to hospital and posthospital care, to nursing home care, and most recently, to annual wellness visits and chronic disease management. DispatchHealth's value proposition is being welcomed by investors, partners, and patients. It has expanded into fifty markets across thirty-four states and raised over $600 million since its founding ten years ago.

Let me share one other example of this expansion across the continuum of care. In 2015 Dr. Renee Dua, a former nephrologist, formed Heal, a home care company, with her entrepreneur-engineer husband, Nick Desai. More recently, in 2021 they created Renee, a care concierge service to help older and underserved Americans to coordinate, communicate, and connect all aspects of their healthcare. During my podcast interview with this power couple, they provided some brilliant insights into how our thinking needs to be reframed to get past the notion that only medical buildings can provide the setting to properly treat patients at the level of care they require. Here are some of Renee's thoughts:

> I'll say, as a nephrologist, my patients who did the best, who always outlived their diagnosis and felt empowered, were those who were doing dialysis at home. They had very involved caretakers and partners. And it really turned the light on for me—why isn't everything happening at home? To this day, I fundamentally believe that there is no magic that happens inside a [medical] building. I think the best doctors want to spend time with their patients, and it's better to do that in the home. It's not just safer, but patients sleep in their own beds, they wake up in

their own homes, they eat what they want, their caretakers look out for them. All the supplies are there, and the patient has full control of this part of their life.

Heal experienced explosive growth in 2022, expanding by 60 percent and tripling their number of PCPs.[57] Renee, the company, is also witnessing rapid growth. And there are numerous other home-based care offerings that have come onto the scene in the past couple of years. One is Patina Health, a senior-focused primary care company that makes the home the primary site of care. They're being led by veteran healthcare executive Jack Stoddard and were able to raise $50 million of funding in their first year.[58] Here's Jack's point of view: "We also believe that if you are going to make healthcare more personalized and accessible, it should be delivered where people want to be—in their home."[59]

These new companies aren't a mere blip in the healthcare industry. They are the rapidly emerging future of healthcare delivery. Technology is enabling this shift, and it's being funded by health insurance companies, large pharmacy chains, and venture capital (VC). Not only are they all investing in these companies, but they are also partnering with them and, in some cases, even acquiring them. We'll discuss the "titans of disruption" in chapter 9, but the fact is that the large healthcare insurance companies, megaretailers, and pharmacy chains are all jumping into the home care ecosystem in a big way.

---

57 "Heal Experiences 60% Growth following Annual Enrollment Period," Cision PR Newswire, February 8, 2022, https://www.prnewswire.com/news-releases/heal-experiences-60-growth-following-annual-enrollment-period-301476950.html.

58 John George, "Patina Reaches Medicare Advantage Plan Deals with 3 Major Insurers to Expand Philadelphia Reach," *Philadelphia Business Journal*, December 21, 2022, https://www.bizjournals.com/philadelphia/news/2022/12/21/patina-aetna-cigna-united-healthcare-medicare.html.

59 "One Year of Profoundly Transforming the Healthcare and Aging Experience," Patina, February 22, 2023, https://patinahealth.com/one-year-of-profoundly-transforming-the-healthcare-and-aging-experience/.

For now, let's wrap up part I of this book, which highlighted the megatrends that are revolutionizing healthcare delivery. As we've discovered, these megatrends are getting beyond the walls in a very literal way, shifting from within hospital and clinic walls to decentralized sites of care, including our homes. In part II, we'll look at some humanistic movements that are changing how we conceive of and receive healthcare. And we'll transition from a concrete and literal take on beyond the walls to one that involves conceptual transformations.

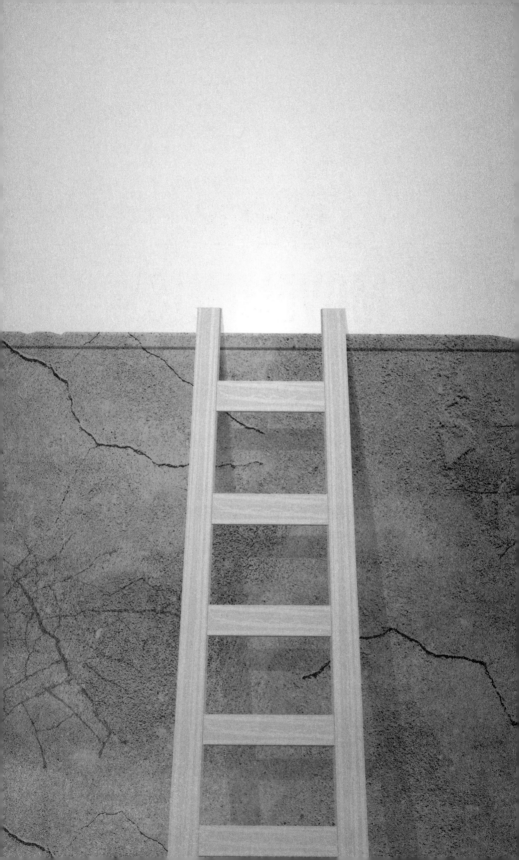

PART II

MOVEMENTS

I am done watching colleagues and communities suffer and die at the expense of what others would just consider an inconvenience. And I just am tired of watching the same community members suffer the same reality, when those who are in power are blind to the entire equation.
–Michellene Davis, Esq., president of the National Medical Fellowship, Inc.

IN PART I, WE DISCUSSED the megatrends emerging from beyond the walls that are transforming the landscape of healthcare. We covered (1) the enabling power of digital and analytic technologies, (2) the shift in the point of care to the point of need, and (3) the transposition of care from the brick-and-mortar healthcare delivery system to a home-based care ecosystem.

In part II, we go beyond *trends* to what I'll call "humanistic healthcare *movements*." Like most movements, they hold the potential for significant disruption. It's my belief that these movements will introduce much-needed ethical transformation into our current systems. The humanistic movements we will discuss are as follows:

1. **The senior care movement**: This movement is focused on the unprecedented number of seniors who will be needing care in the coming decades and how we can leverage a combination of technology and empathy to address their needs.

2. **The contextual care movement**: This is a movement focused on how we must approach patient care with a deeper understanding of the significant impact of peoples' day-to-day lives on healthcare outcomes.

3. **The "whole person" health movement**: This movement focuses on how we must go beyond treating clinical ailments and widen our aperture to focus on the patient's overall emotional, relational, and spiritual health.

Part II of the book highlights three specific humanistic healthcare movements that are truly 'beyond the walls' initiatives, but there are many more I do not have the space to cover. These include but are not limited to the behavioral health movement; the substance dependency movement; the women's health movement; the LGBTQ+ healthcare movement; the climate change/global warming and sustainability healthcare movement; the rural health movement; the SDOH movement; the lifestyle, wellness, and integrative medicine movements; and the disparities, equity, and inclusion healthcare movements. Each of these movements could easily occupy a complete chapter, if not a book. Each is important from a clinical, ethical, economic, and public health perspective. As one example of the economic imperative, a report from Deloitte projects that the US healthcare system could save hundreds of billions of dollars over the next few years by making healthcare more equitable. As the report demonstrates, inequities in the US health system cost approximately *$320 billion today* and could eclipse *$1 trillion* in annual spending by 2040 if left unaddressed. The report states that this situation is "signaling an unsustainable crisis for the industry."[60] The overarching point here is that these humanistic movements are not optional if we are to optimize and sustain the health of all Americans now and for the next few generations. They are not ancillary "social responsibility" add-ons to the important work at hand. They are, in fact, fundamental to healthcare.

I had the privilege of interviewing Michellene Davis in 2021. Ms. Davis is an accomplished lawyer and currently the CEO of the National Medical Fellowship, Inc. Michellene previously served as the executive vice president and chief corporate affairs officer at RWJBarn-abas Health, the largest academic medical center system in New Jersey. And prior to that, she served as chief policy counsel to former New Jersey governor Jon Corzine. Ms. Davis was the first African American to serve in this position and the first African American to serve as acting New Jersey state treasurer, responsible for a state budget of over $30 billion. Toward the end of our interview, I ask Michellene why she upended her brilliant career to shift to a nonprofit focused on raising educational funds for minority medical students. Her response was the most eloquent and moving I've ever heard on the urgency of these humanistic movements in healthcare. Here is a snippet of what she shared and a thought to keep in mind as we make our way through the next several chapters:

At the height of the pandemic, I watched no fewer than thirty of my colleagues perish. And when you look at who perished and who are the most vulnerable in our communities ... well, after

---

60 Neal Batra et al., "U.S. Health Care Can't Afford Health Inequities," *Deloitte Insights*, June 22, 2022, https://www2.deloitte.com/us/en/insights/industry/health-care/economic-cost-of-health-disparities.html.

that I just realized that we are done dying. I am done watching colleagues and communities suffer and die at the expense of what others would just consider an inconvenience. And I am tired of watching the same community members suffer the same reality, when those who are in power are blind to the entire equation. And for me, what shifted was that on this side of COVID, with whatever amount of time I might have left on this planet ... I needed every second of it to truly matter, to address this one ill, to save even one life, and to change the face of medicine.

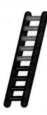

CHAPTER 4

THE CARE OF THE ELDERLY

There are a lot of older adults, and there are
not enough people to care for them.
–Andrew Parker, founder and CEO of Papa

We need to rethink how we treat seniors, especially since we are witnessing a massive shift into that demographic that will continue for decades. The aging of our society is much larger and will last much longer than most people realize. The Advisory Board, a healthcare think tank, put together some startling facts and figures, including some of the challenges seniors will face:

- In 2010 no baby boomer had yet turned sixty-five. At this point in time and into the foreseeable future, **over ten thousand Americans will turn sixty-five every single day.**

- Projections indicate that **by 2060 there will be roughly ninety-five million people over sixty-five in the United States compared with fifty-six million in 2023.**

- Isolation is a growing problem. **Older people are more likely to live alone** in the United States than anywhere else in the world.

- **From 1999 to 2019, there was a 543 percent increase in total debt for Americans over age seventy**, the largest percentage increase for any age group.

- Future seniors will be less likely to have pensions and adequate retirement savings compared with previous generations. **By 2029 over half of middle-income older adults will not be able to afford to live in senior living facilities.**

- **Life expectancy continues to rise in the United States**, which, combined with the fact that there will be more people over sixty-five than ever before, will put an unprecedented strain on our healthcare system—and could potentially even bankrupt it.[61]

- **Eighty percent of Americans over sixty-five years of age already have a chronic disease, and 68 percent have two or more.** In addition, the over sixty-five demographic has double-digit percentages of Alzheimer's disease and dementia, kidney disease, and depression.[62]

In 2034 America will reach a new milestone. That year, the US Census Bureau projects that older adults will edge out children in population size. People aged sixty-five and over are expected to number 77 million, while children under age eighteen will number

---

61   Miriam Sznycer-Taub, "Caring for an Aging Population: Past, Present, Future," Advisory Board, March 28, 2022, https://www.advisory.com/topics/strategy-planning-and-growth/2022/03/caring-for-an-aging-population-infographic.

62   "The Top 10 Most Common Chronic Conditions in Older Adults," National Council on Aging, April 23, 2021, https://www.ncoa.org/article/the-top-10-most-common-chronic-conditions-in-older-adults.

76.5 million.[63] As the sixty-five-plus population grows to these peak numbers, the costs of care in the United States will skyrocket.

According to the Kaiser Family Foundation, Medicare currently provides health insurance coverage for about a fifth of our population, about sixty-five million people. That spending comprises 12 percent of the federal budget and 20 percent of overall national healthcare spending. From 2000 to 2021 alone, Medicare benefit payments rose from $200 billion to $689 billion, translating to an average annual growth rate of 6.2 percent. In addition, annual Medicare spending per person also grew from 2000 to 2021, increasing from $5,800 to $15,300. Projections indicate that by 2032, net Medicare outlays will cost nearly *$1.6 trillion* due to growth both in the number of Medicare patients as well as the increased costs associated with a greater number of chronic conditions.[64] By then Medicare expenses will take up almost 6 percent of our country's GDP.

Medicare (as well as Medicaid) was created back in 1965 during President Johnson's administration when they realized that seniors often lacked the financial resources to secure and pay for proper healthcare toward the end of their lives. I say "toward the end of their lives" because in 1965, American men were expected to live to sixty-seven and American women to seventy-four. So in essence, Medicare was a federally sponsored end-of-life healthcare payment plan preventing individuals and their families from accumulating huge amounts of medical debt in the last years of their life. The original version of Medicare could not account for the much longer life spans and the greater chronic care health needs of older adults today. At the present

---

63   Jonathan Vespa, "The U.S. Joins Other Countries with Large Aging Populations," US Census, March 13, 2018, https://www.census.gov/library/stories/2018/03/graying-america.html.

64   "The Facts about Medicare Spending," Kaiser Family Foundation, June 2022, https://www.kff.org/interactive/medicare-spending/.

time, American men are expected to live to seventy-six and American women to eighty-one.[65]

In 1997 the Medicare Advantage program (Part C of Medicare) was introduced partly to alleviate the cost escalations of the traditional FFS model. The Advantage program was expanded in 2003, and in 2006 Medicare Part D became law, providing seniors with prescription drug benefits. All of these revisions were designed to address the limitations of the FFS payment and to support seniors being taken care of by local health maintenance organizations, which would receive a monthly per-patient fee in order to provide care that was more continuous and more comprehensive.

Despite these changes in payment, a fundamental problem remains. Our American healthcare system is not designed for aging seniors. It's not customized or adapted for many of the unique issues and challenges seniors face. To be blunt, the system is inadequate. This opinion is largely shared by healthcare policy and public health experts, as well as the gerontologists and geriatricians who care for seniors.

> Our American healthcare system is not designed for aging seniors.

Speaking of geriatricians, there are currently about 7,300 in the United States. These are physicians who have specialized training in the care of the elderly, including the frail elderly. That's not nearly enough. That's about 1 geriatrician for every 10,000 seniors in our country. It's estimated that by 2030 we will need roughly 33,000 geriatricians,

---

65   "Table V.A4.—Period Life Expectancy," *2022 OASDI Trustees Report*, Social Security Administration, accessed March 23, 2023, https://www.ssa.gov/oact/TR/2022/lr5a4.html.

but we will probably only have about a fifth of that number.[66] That should strike all of us as a disturbing shortfall.

What we know is that geriatricians, because of their training and experience, do a better job addressing senior health, including palliative care, hospice care, nursing home care, and cognitive care. They have special expertise in knowing what combination of medications the elderly should avoid because of health risks and side effects. Given their unique knowledge and experience, geriatricians provide better outcomes for seniors than other primary care doctors. For example, a 2021 study from the UK showed lowered hospital lengths of stay and lowered costs when senior patients were cared for by geriatricians compared with other doctors.[67] Decreasing the ratio of geriatricians to senior patients will strain our healthcare system and become a significant problem for seniors, their families, and for all of us taxpayers who will be financing Medicare.

Humana has been aware of these challenges and has been making multibillion-dollar acquisitions and investments in senior care over the past several years. Part of that investment includes establishing senior care clinics. They've already created over 220 of them and expect to double that number by 2025.[68] These clinics are designed to transcend the limitations of general primary care as well as FFS payment models by enabling providers to customize their care and have the time and resources required to care for older patients.

Because these clinics are funded by Medicare Advantage, doctors receive a certain payment each month for each patient. As

66   "The Physician Shortage in Geriatrics," ChenMed, March 18, 2022, https://www. chenmed.com/blog/physician-shortage-geriatrics.

67   Reshma Aziz Merchant et al., "Outcomes of Care by Geriatricians and Non-Geriatricians in an Academic Hospital," *Frontiers in Medicine* 9 (June 6, 2022): 908100, https://doi.org/10.3389/fmed.2022.908100.

68   "Investor Day Presentation 2022," Humana, September 15, 2022, https://humana. gcs-web.com/static-files/aed79f8e-2b14-4891-a76f-d20e58303212.

a result, the financial incentive to see more patients per day is greatly lessened. That allows doctors to spend more time per patient and to provide care in more cost-effective ways. Those monthly Medicare Advantage payments also allow providers to invest in a multidisciplinary team for their senior patients, which might include pharmacists, social workers, health coaches, and behaviorists, as well as transportation and social services.

Over the past few years, we've seen entrepreneurial provider groups and, more recently, legacy stakeholders begin to redesign care to ensure that it is customized for seniors. These are 'beyond the walls' thinkers who, through their innovative start-ups and initiatives, have inspired this growing movement. You're about to meet three whose ideas have already triggered buy-in from the big healthcare players.

BRINGING IT HOME: MIKE LE

Dr. Mike Le is a dedicated physician and entrepreneur. He cofounded Landmark Health, which has successfully brought a revolutionary senior home-based care model into the mainstream. Their approach combines the ideas from the last section—tech-enabled care brought into the patients' home when patients need it—plus a highly customized and personalized focus on seniors.

Mike was inspired by his father, who was a physician with a general medical practice in a small town in Massachusetts. Believe it or not, Mike's father still made house calls, carrying his little black bag to various home visits. Mike grew up seeing the tremendous positive impact his dad had on his patients by coming to care for them where they lived. He also saw how doing so provided his father with a much better understanding of the patients he served, in a way that would be nearly impossible in a medical office setting.

From that firm foundation, Mike brought the best of the past to bear on the present, creating a hi-tech, high-touch, team-based model that delivers state-of-the-art care in the comfort, convenience, and safety of the older patient's home. The care model is intensive, offering blood tests, X-rays, ultrasounds, IVs, catheter placements, wound care, and suturing. This type of care would be welcomed by anyone, but it's especially appreciated by senior patients with complex chronic conditions and end-stage diseases as well as those seniors with debilitating conditions, such as dementia and frailty. Mike shared with me during a podcast interview, "When we tell our patients what we offer, and they experience it for themselves, they often tell us that it's almost too good to be true."

Landmark's 'beyond the walls' vision is now embedded in mainstream healthcare. Landmark grew to cover 250,000 patients across twenty states and was then acquired in 2021 by Optum Health, a care provider owned by UnitedHealthcare. It's now an integral part of Optum's large Home and Community division, the vision for which, Mike went on to say, "is to break down silos and improve collaboration, to give patients a seamless care experience across their entire continuum of needs." Their goal, according to Mike, is to expand and scale the business across the country, and it's well on its way. Landmark's home-based medical care model now covers over half a million seniors and grew 30 percent year over year between 2019 and 2022.[69] Landmark focuses on the top 8 to 10 percent of patients who are homebound and would have tremendous difficulty getting to their doctor. This relative minority of patients probably accounts for over half the total Medicare costs.

---

69   "Provider Groups Turn to Landmark to Effectively Extend High-Touch, In-Home Medical Care to High Utilizers," Landmark Health, July 28, 2022, https://www.landmarkhealth.org/resource/provider-groups-turn-to-landmark-to-effectively-extend-high-touch-in-home-medical-care-to-high-utilizers/.

One of the things I so admire about Mike and his colleagues is their mission and integrity. The following are his own words:

We didn't start with the financial model. We said, "Okay, let's start with the patient." When we looked at it, we saw we would need a very large and expensive team to deliver comprehensive care in the homes. How do we finance that? The only way was through risk-bearing contracts and being able to partner with health plans to deliver this care on a capitated [payment] basis. That was the genesis. We would start with the patient first and then figure out the finances and how to deliver the care model without compromising on all of the specific pieces that we thought would drive value for these sick and frail seniors.

Similar to Raphael Rakowski, Mike and his Landmark colleagues developed the following pillars to create a new ecosystem of care in the home, this time specifically based on seniors' needs:

Pillar 1: Realizing that a Monday through Friday, nine-to-five model wasn't going to meet the needs of these patients, Landmark decided on 24/7 care.

Pillar 2: Understanding that over 50 percent of these patients have profound unidentified psychosocial challenges, Landmark decided to embed the SDOH into their model by identifying nonclinical needs such as food, shopping and meal prep, financial assistance, housing issues, travel, and social isolation. And because in traditional healthcare settings, it can take weeks to months to see a behavioral health specialist, the company decided to bring that service in-house and make it a part of its multidisciplinary team. In fact, the very first physician Mike hired was a psychiatrist.

Pillar 3: As a longtime practicing hospitalist, Mike has repeatedly witnessed how poorly end-of-life conversations happen in the hospital setting—often in the last minutes of a patient's ED or ICU stay. So Landmark made palliative care training a requirement for its providers and teams.

Pillar 4: Given that many senior patients are on multiple complicated medication regimens, Landmark made sure that a pharmacist was embedded in each of the teams.

Pillar 5: Given that the time after hospital or nursing home discharge can be a very fragile period in patients' lives, Landmark arranged frequent touch points within the first thirty days after discharge as well as highly protocolized team coordination.

Mike and his colleagues have expanded the horizons of what home care can be for an aging population. They've designed it, deployed it, and committed the resources to sustain it. They've adopted a viable business model through Medicare Advantage payment and worked with provider groups and insurance companies to support and sustain it. Again, what motivates Mike and his colleagues is not so much the financials as that this customized care for seniors is demonstrably better care. Again, here are his own words:

My favorite stat at Landmark came from when we looked at fifteen thousand patients who were receiving the Landmark care and then compared them to fifteen thousand patients similarly matched across multiple factors but not receiving care from Landmark. We found that there was a 26 percent reduction in mortality for the patients that we were treating! I do think that so much of healthcare is coming to the home, as well as this holistic, proactive, preventative model of care that has the urgent capabilities to stabilize in place.

Hopefully, it will become the standard of care someday for those patients who are the sickest and most frail.

ENDING SENIOR LONELINESS: ANDREW PARKER

While Dr. Mike Le and his colleagues were bringing an all-encompassing vision for senior home-based care, Andrew Parker was seeking a solution for a specific, widespread, and devastating problem for the elderly—loneliness and social isolation.

Andrew began his company, Papa, in response to his real-life grandfather experiencing those very issues. Andrew rightfully realized that if his own "Papa" was experiencing problems related to companionship, assistance, and transportation, many other seniors were as well. Andrew said, "He needed assistance. He was lonely and isolated. He didn't have a car and wasn't able to drive, but he didn't need bathing and toileting. So the traditional services didn't make a lot of sense for him."

How serious is living with loneliness and social isolation? And does it impact one's health? According to the National Institute on Aging, research has linked social isolation and loneliness to higher risks for a variety of physical and mental conditions such as high blood pressure, heart disease, obesity, weakened immune system, anxiety, depression, cognitive decline, Alzheimer's disease, and even death.[70] A recent book summarizing over eight decades of research in the Harvard Study of Adult Development notes that lonely people live shorter lives and that chronic loneliness increases a person's odds of

---

70   John T. Cacioppo and Stephanie Cacioppo, "Older Adults Reporting Social Isolation or Loneliness Show Poorer Cognitive Function 4 Years Later," *Evidence-Based Nursing* 17, no. 2 (April 2014): 59–60, https://doi.org/10.1136/eb-2013-101379.

death, in any given year, by 26 percent.[71] In other words, the answer is a resounding yes. Loneliness and social isolation are indeed real health problems—more like a silent epidemic that is harming and shortening the lives of tens of millions of Americans.

In fact, according to another study from Harvard, 36 percent of adult Americans report feeling "serious loneliness." For clarification, this malady extends beyond seniors and includes individuals of all ages and demographics.[72]

> The Harvard Study of Adult Development notes that lonely people live shorter lives and that chronic loneliness increases a person's odds of death, in any given year, by 26 percent.

Loneliness is an international health crisis as well. In Great Britain, the government has appointed a "minister of loneliness" to address what has become a major public health challenge. The magnitude of this public health hazard in the United States is so large and so concerning that the US general surgeon Dr. Vivek Murthy wrote an entire book dedicated to it—*Together: The Healing Power of Human Connection in a Sometimes Lonely World*—in which he compares the harmful impact of loneliness to smoking half a pack of cigarettes per day.[73]

What's shocking is that, prior to Papa, no one had ever come up with a scalable and sustainable approach to addressing these issues. Andrew's "beyond the wall" solution is uniquely empathetic, tech-

---

71   Robert Waldinger and Marc Schulz, *The Good Life: Lessons from the World's Longest Scientific Study of Happiness* (New York: Simon & Schuster, 2023).

72   Richard Weissbourd et al., "Loneliness in America: How the Pandemic Has Deepened an Epidemic of Loneliness and What We Can Do About It," Harvard Graduate School of Education, Making Caring Common Project, October 2020, https://mcc.gse.harvard.edu/reports/loneliness-in-america.

73   Vivek Murthy, *Together: The Healing Power of Human Connection in a Sometimes Lonely World* (New York: Harper Wave, 2020).

enabled, scalable, and affordable. It's another great example of how the digital era, the shift to home-based care, and a customized focus on this segment of the population can transform lives.

Like Mike, Andrew didn't create his company just to make a living. He created it out of empathy after he discovered that the traditional healthcare services didn't work for seniors. It turned out to be a solution that healthcare consumers and investors really value. In November 2021 Papa was valued at $1.4 billion, raising $150 million in series D funding and bringing its total funding to $250 million since its founding in 2017.

There's another critically important point I discovered in speaking to Andrew, which resonates with Raphael Rakowski's success factor in scaling the hospital-at-home model. The key, according to both Andrew and Raphael, is tech-enabled logistics. I suspect that the details are probably quite boring to most of us, but it's the secret sauce almost every entrepreneur I've spoken to has revealed. Andrew was an early employee at MDLIVE, one of the largest telehealth companies, where he ran strategy, product development, and sales and brought a tech-enabled platform to over thirty million Americans. What he learned in that role was how to scale care delivery from a mom-and-pop manual operation to a highly automated logistics platform, greatly reducing the inefficiencies and substantially lowering the costs. From an operational, tech, and business perspective, we should view this as a brilliant move, but I also view it from an expanded humanistic and medical lens and believe that Andrew does too. Andrew said, "Loneliness is an epidemic among seniors. Just think about an eighty-year-old sitting on the couch for weeks at a time, maybe months, maybe years, with very little to no human interaction—and just think about the negative effects created."

From a financial standpoint, Papa is covered by Medicare benefits and through large commercial insurers—that's, in part, due to Andrew and his colleagues having demonstrated that it works. Their services are currently available through sixty-five health plans: "Most of our business is distributed through large health insurance companies, where this is actually free to the older adult and paid for by the health plan. And [the insurance companies] don't pay for things just because they're nice to have. It's the fact that this actually improves health-care outcomes, reduces overall costs, and has all these other positive effects on one's life. We've seen that by pairing a "Papa Pal" with an older adult, we're able to reduce emergency department visits, reduce hospital readmissions, and improve medication adherence."

At the start, most Papa Pals were college students, but Andrew has discovered that a lot of other older adults, including retirees, want to do this type of work. Through the Papa app, Papa Pals are matched with a senior who wants the service and can set up an appointment to spend a couple of hours per week at the senior's home. (The average visit is two and a half hours.) Andrew has also automated the rigorous process of screening the Papa Pals.

One other critical success factor built into Andrew's approach is consumer obsession. The Silicon Valley entrepreneurs call this "10x." When you create digital tech, you have to strive to be ten times better than a nondigital product in delivering a convenient, easy-to-use, and valuable experience. Through the Papa app, seniors get to rate their Papa Pals, and the Papa Pals keep a record of who they've visited, what they did, how long they were there, and other basic details. If there is a health problem with a senior, Papa Pals will notify the doctor's office of that person and get them timely assistance. Papa Pals are not clinicians, and they do not offer any medical advice or clinical care.

But as Andrew will tell you, they definitely do a lot of other things that we now know have an outsize impact on health outcomes.

What they will do is take you to the doctor, go grocery shopping with you, teach you how to use an iPhone, play a game of canasta with you, even write down your life story. They'll do anything that I was doing for my grandfather. They're an extension of your family and a representation of a grandchild. We had a member yesterday say that they wish they could win the lotto so that they could get a Papa Pal every day. To hear that from an older person, it really hits you. To hear a member say, "I stopped taking Xanax, and I don't feel I have to go to my therapist anymore because my main issue was that I was just alone. I needed someone to be a friend," I'm very proud of that.

A SENIOR CONCIERGE SERVICE ON STEROIDS: CHRIS CHEN

Dr. Chris Chen and his physician brother, Gordon, were highly motivated by their father's health saga to find a solution for the lack of accountability they observed in our healthcare system. ChenMed, the start-up begun by Chris and his family, tackles that problem head-on. ChenMed is a highly successful senior care practice, now spanning dozens of cities across numerous states. It's been recognized for its groundbreaking care model by the White House, the Department of Health and Human Services (HHS), and the UK National Health System. *Medical Economics* named ChenMed "the best primary care system in the U.S.," and *Fortune* magazine named ChenMed one of its "Change the World" companies in 2020.[74] Chris, cofounder and CEO of ChenMed, began his professional career as an Ivy League–trained cardiologist. He could have been hugely successful in that career path. Instead, because of what he saw happen with his father's care, he chose to tackle senior care instead. This strong ethical bent and the segmented, customized approach are something that were also inspired by his father, who had a thriving Miami-based senior care practice for many years prior to ChenMed. Chris is yet another example of entrepreneurs driven by a humanistic mission and personal commitment: "The number one thing that my dad taught me when I was growing up was, 'Chris, if you want to make a good living, you don't go after making a good living. Do the right things, and the money will come. And apply all of your efforts to that.'"

Chris and the entire Chen family discerned very early on that the American healthcare system was not designed, organized, or resourced to provide appropriate, humane care for elderly patients, especially those with complex situations and those who are poor.[75]

Having understood this decades ago, the Chens created what Chris refers to as "a concierge service on steroids," one that, "substantially improves health, substantially reduces hospitalizations, and minimizes extremely expensive and debilitating catastrophic events."

Similar to Medically Home and Landmark, ChenMed's approach is built on several fundamentals.

With ChenMed, the number of patients each doctor cares for is markedly reduced so that the doctors and their teams can spend a lot more time with patients both during visits and in between visits.

---

74 "About ChenMed," ChenMed, accessed March 23, 2023, https://www.chenmed.com/news/chenmed-model-transforms-healthcare-and-provides-much-needed-support-seniors.

75 Christopher Chen and Gordon Chen, *The Calling: A Memoir of Family, Faith, and the Future of Healthcare* (Nashville: Forefront Books, 2022).

While a typical physician-to-patient ratio could be 1,700:1,[76] at ChenMed it's approximately 400 patients to each care team. Second, the frequency of visits is monthly, as opposed to three or four times a year. Third, while traditional healthcare has finally realized the importance of the nonclinical or SDOH and the importance of psychosocial factors such as loneliness, ChenMed understood this years ago and created its own transportation service to bring patients to the clinic as well as set up social gatherings in its medical buildings after hours: "We don't just do the medical stuff. We do centers in which we're doing activities like line or salsa dancing. So there is a whole socialization aspect of it. My father, who has a master's degree, a PhD, and an MD, came to me the other day and said, 'Chris, I am not sure what has a larger impact, the amazing clinical care or when our patients come to our centers, when we smile, we hug, and we love on them.'"

The Chens understood that in order to offer a superior clinical service, they needed an integrated platform from which to operate it, and so they built one. Let me be clear: they didn't build another onerous electronic medical record system. They built a customized care platform to enable doctors and their teams to provide up-to-date, evidence-based, highly reliable, and standardized care. While most electronic medical records get in the way of providers practicing relationally focused medicine, the ChenMed platform does the opposite—it supports it. The platform is so critical that ChenMed built a stand-alone, award-winning tech company to develop and continuously update its digital care platform.

According to Chris and Gordon, doctors need to adopt a different mindset, one that's more humanistic and holistic. When ChenMed brings in new physicians, the company puts them through a crash

---

76   Jonathan P. Weiner, "Prepaid Group Practice Staffing and U.S. Physician Supply: Lessons for Workforce Policy," *Health Affairs* (Project HOPE) Suppl Web Exclusives (2004): W4-43-59, https://doi.org/10.1377/hlthaff.w4.43.

course—it's not surprising that Chris refers to it as a "brainwashing" course. The company spends around six months retraining their providers to think differently and to practice differently. They take this retraining so seriously that if a doctor doesn't pass this bootcamp, that person gets booted.

The Chens aren't joking around. They take the cultural, emotional, and relational part of healthcare seriously. Per Chris, "See, what you have to do, you have to fundamentally change the mindset of the caregivers. We're not trained to be held accountable for the actual outcome for a patient while almost every other industry in America is held accountable for results. That's a huge fundamental shift in healthcare—the concept of accountability."

From a business model and financial accountability perspective, ChenMed, like Landmark, is based on Medicare Advantage payments. The business gets paid on a per-member, per-month basis—no matter if the patient comes to the clinic or not and no matter how many or how few tests and procedures they order. In sharp contrast to an FFS payment model, ChenMed has no financial incentive to do more than is required or to try to force its doctors to see scores of patients per day. That also means that any savings generated from lower hospital admission rates, which ChenMed consistently achieves, can be used to pay for increased levels of preventive care and smaller patient panels.

During and in the aftermath of the pandemic, that was an incredibly sound business model—a sort of "ark" during the torrential financial crisis that most primary care and specialty practices as well as hospitals encountered. According to analysis from the Kaiser Family Foundation, physician visits dropped 14 percent from Q1 2020 to Q2 of the same year. In late 2022 patient visit numbers had recovered but still lagged behind prepandemic levels. Hospital discharges followed similar patterns, dropping 16 percent in March

2020 without having returned to 2019 levels.[77] For the majority of practices and hospital systems, this decline in utilization meant a drastic reduction in revenue.

To maintain access to healthcare and to support FFS-based hospitals and providers, the federal government instituted a public health emergency waiver, part of which provided payment for virtual visits at parity with in-person visits. But even with that bit of aid, we witnessed tremendous financial losses and saw hundreds of practices shutter their doors. Given ChenMed's Medicare Advantage payment model, they could easily temper the storm of reduced visits because they continued to receive their monthly capitation payments. It's no surprise that they've seen consistent growth over the past few years and, more recently, even more accelerated multistate expansion. Since its founding, ChedMed has seen 35 percent average annual growth with nearly one hundred medical centers in over twenty cities and twelve states. They were the only healthcare company named to Fortune's "Change the World" list in 2020.[78]

Entrepreneurs who have taken a humanistic stand to create a completely different and transformative approach to healthcare delivery for seniors in our country are inspiring, and their work is hard to do. These 'beyond the walls' solutions are by no means perfect, but they demonstrate the potential power of identifying a genuine need and bringing to bear the full breadth of a consumer-first approach to solving it. In the next chapters, we'll encounter two other humanistic movements in healthcare that deploy system-wide, tech-enabled shifts to contextualized, whole-person care.

77 Matthew McGough, Krutika Amin, and Cynthia Cox, "How Has Healthcare Utilization Changed since the Pandemic?" Health System Tracker, Kaiser Family Foundation, January 23, 2023, https://www.healthsystemtracker.org/chart-collection/how-has-healthcare-utilization-changed-since-the-pandemic/.

78 "ChenMed: InFocus," ChenMed, 2019, https://www.chenmed.com/sites/default/files/2022-09/InFocus.pdf.

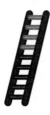

CHAPTER 5

THE RISE OF CONTEXTUAL CARE

Recovery is everyone's problem and no one's job.
—Yoni Shtein, CEO and cofounder, Laguna Health

ontextual care concerns are nonclinical healthcare issues that have a demonstrable and immediate impact on individuals' health outcomes. While there is some overlap with the SDOH, contextual concerns are broader in scope. The CDC defines SDOH as "the conditions in the environments where people are born, live, learn, work, play, worship, and age that affect a wide range of health, functioning, and quality-of-life outcomes and risks."[79] I tend to think of the SDOH as macro factors and the contextual ones as a set of *personalized* SDOH factors. The contextual factors we'll be discussing in this chapter were derived from nearly two decades of in-depth analysis of dialogues between patients and providers.

---

79   "Social Determinants of Health," Healthy People 2030, US Department of Health and Human Services Office of Disease Prevention and Health Promotion, accessed March 24, 2023, https://health.gov/healthypeople/priority-areas/social-determinants-health.

Because we use the words "nonclinical" and "nonmedical," there is the temptation to dismiss contextual care as an optional add-on to traditional healthcare, akin to buying a nicer model car that has a sunroof, heated seats, etc. In other words, nice to have but not necessary. But that's just not the case.

For many people, contextual issues can be the root cause that, when serious enough, adversely impacts outcomes such as recovery from a hospitalization. Think of someone who just had a major surgery and who has recently lost their spouse. They return to an empty home, not only missing their life partner but also without anyone else in the home to assist them during their recovery period. That's a contextual barrier to recovery. Or think of someone facing difficult financial straits for whom the level of immediate stress (not being able to afford all their medications or healthy food or pay their electricity bill) will impact their recovery and health. Those are contextual barriers to recovery. There are countless examples of patients returning from inpatient settings to not-so-great life circumstances where their state of mind or even their actual physical health is threatened. They're supposed to be recovering but lack the resources to regain wellness. If these types of contextual care issues are not identified and addressed, medical interventions will often not be as successful as they could have been, assuming they don't completely fail.

Two of the outstanding trailblazers we'll spotlight in this chapter are Dr. Saul Weiner, who, along with his partner, Dr. Alan Schwartz, has devoted almost twenty years to studying the effects of contextual care as well as the devastating effects of ignoring them. Saul and Alan actually coined the term "contextual care." They created the approach and continue to expand it in their work with Laguna Health. For the past two decades, Saul and Alan have been working within the physical walls of traditional healthcare but elevating their thinking beyond those walls. Their clinical work and research were all accomplished within the Veterans Health Affairs (VHA) system. They're demonstrating what it looks like to transcend walls by bringing their learnings from a traditional system to a start-up that is anything but traditional and then bringing their experience in Laguna Health back into traditional hospital systems.

When I first heard their story during our podcast interview, it completely resonated with my own. It took me back to the first decade of my career when I was seeing patients and teaching internal medicine residents and medical students. In my first year as an attending physician, I saw an older gentleman, probably close to seventy years old at the time. He was Black and lived in the Bronx. We eventually became quite close, but our first visit together was rocky.

During that first encounter, I discovered that his blood pressure wasn't controlled, his cholesterol was abnormal, his blood sugar was also high, and he was a little overweight. I asked if he exercised, and he said no. I asked if he ate lots of fruits and vegetables, and he said no. My training within the traditional clinical framework took over. I launched into a lecture about the risks of high blood pressure, high cholesterol, high blood sugar, and being overweight. And I recommended that he find a gym and start exercising regularly. I also recommended that he stop buying processed, high-carb foods and begin purchasing vegetables and fruits instead and eating lean proteins. He sat silently as I spoke. In fact, I remember admiring his demeanor. He had a silent wisdom about him.

What I didn't realize was that he was about to share that wisdom with me—in a pretty blunt way. After I finished my minilecture, I sat back and waited for his response. He leaned forward and began a lesson that would change the course of my thinking and my career. "Son ... Doctor ... do you know where I live? Do you know what my neighborhood is like? Do you know how much money I have to spend? Do you know what my apartment looks like or who I live with, or anything else for that matter? What do you actually know about me before you begin telling me what I need to do?" It was a rhetorical question because he and I both knew that I knew almost nothing about him or his life. He went on, "I'll bet you live in Manhattan, probably the Upper East Side. You have a lovely apartment, and I'll bet you have a gym membership right in your neighborhood. I'll also venture to say that you have a few upscale groceries within easy walking distance of your apartment. Am I right?"

I sheepishly replied, "Yes, that's right. All of it is right."

He nodded with no evidence of satisfaction on his face and continued, "Well, I'm going to tell you where I live. I live a few blocks from here. My apartment is a studio. It's small and cramped. I live alone now that my wife has passed. We never had children, so it's pretty lonely. The stove used to work when my wife was alive, but it doesn't now, and I don't have the money to replace it. So I mostly cook off of a small electric hot pot. There are no groceries in my neighborhood with fresh foods. I can get some stuff, mostly from the bodegas nearby. And by the way, it's not like I can go somewhere and grab bags of fresh food. The gangs here in this section of the Bronx are mean. If I go out and they see me going to the market, they know I'm carrying cash, and I'm an easy target. If I walk back to the apartment with bags, they know I have food and probably cash—again, an easy target. So I try to buy as little as possible at a time instead of carrying grocery bags. I'm just trying to survive my neighborhood and survive with the little money I get from the government. As for a gym, do you see a fancy gym anywhere here in this neighborhood? The only exercise I get is walking fast so I don't get mugged. So listen. I can tell you're a good person and a good doctor, and you mean well. And I'm sure you're going to do a lot of good in your career—help a lot of people. But can I give you one piece of advice? Why don't you find out more about a person before you tell them what they should be doing?"

That patient, that moment, that advice changed everything for me.

I began asking other doctors, including the residents I was training, if they were asking their patients questions about the context of their lives. I also began sitting in and observing other doctors as they saw their patients, hoping to learn how they learned about their patients' lives. I scoured the literature and joined academic groups that were focused on studying this issue. We used terms such as "empathy" and "relationship-centered care." This work became the focus of my first decade as a doctor and the theme of my entire career. It defined my professional purpose, which is to humanize healthcare.

> "Why don't you find out more about a person before you tell them what they should be doing?"

As I listened to Saul and Alan tell their story, I was taken right back to my core purpose. You'll understand why as you consider Dr. Weiner's story:

> *I got interested in this almost twenty years ago when I was a junior attending physician supervising patients. I would typically hear about a patient in the back office and then go see the patient with the resident. What I noticed was that the resident would come back and present the patient to me, and it sounded good. They looked everything up, and it seemed like they had a plan, and we'd walk in to see the patient together.*

But often in the conversation with the patient, issues would start to emerge. I'd start to discover there were things going on in that person's life. It could be that they couldn't afford something, or that they had lost a key caregiver, or that they were suddenly responsible for taking care of somebody else who was ill—or it could be something good, like they got a job, and they're working the night shift.

Any of these factors, in the context of the clinical presentation, could be critical. Often, it turned out that what we thought was going to be a good plan just wasn't going to work at all. There was no way that person was going to actually be able to do what we suggested they do, or they weren't going to be able to do it in a way that was going to be safe and effective. And that [contextual] conversation with them led to a revised plan, something that actually did make sense and was going to work for that patient.

After this happened a number of times, I started to think, "Wow, this is a quality-of-care issue. There's something going on here that we don't really have a name for that is critical to getting care right." At that point, we kind of coined the term "contextual error" to describe a situation where a care plan basically looks good on paper. It meets the clinical guidelines. It's based on research evidence. But it's still not the right plan for that person."

I connected with Saul and Alan on so many levels. Like Saul, a part of my first job was teaching residents in training. For the first twelve years of my career, I typically had a couple of teaching clinic sessions a week, and I also oversaw hospital rounds with internal medicine residents in training. I still recall how I would cringe after listening to a patient's story and think to myself, "God, how dehumanizing and how disrespectful our healthcare system is. We're treating people like they're clinical objects. No one's doing anything wrong, but no one's doing things right."

What I didn't have then was a grasp of the concept of contextualized care. I'm excited to see more attention is finally being paid to this important aspect of healthcare. This humanistic movement is only going to become more prominent and powerful in the years to come, and much of that thanks to the professionals you're meeting here.

UNDERSTANDING THE IMPACT OF CONTEXTUAL CARE

Saul and Alan shared numerous real-life examples that helped me understand the clinical impact of contextual care. Their case studies drove home the point that contextual care is an essential part of how our medical system can and should help patients. Consider this case:

An older woman patient was having issues related to not getting dialysis. Instead of showing up for her appointments, she would end up in the emergency room getting dialyzed, where she would be told, "You really need to make your dialysis appointments." Finally, during her fourth ER visit, a medical student asked her what was going on in her life and why she was having trouble getting to her visits. And it turned out that she was taking care of a kid who also needed care but at a different location, and it was not possible for her to simultaneously take care of herself and take care of the kid. She was choosing the child, as many of us might.

Alan went on to share that once the team understood this, they were able to offer the patient dialysis at the same facility where her grandson was receiving his treatments. They were also able to arrange transportation to and from the hospital. The contextual care intervention worked, and she almost never missed a dialysis appointment after that. It had never occurred to her that she could request that change. For any of us who have experienced the bureaucracy of the healthcare system, that's easily understandable.

Pointing out the lack of contextual care is not meant as a criticism of physicians or other providers. It is, however, a critique of our healthcare system. As Saul puts it, doctors are trained to be "efficient task completers" out of the necessities and constraints imposed upon them.

In 2015 Alan and Saul published their landmark book, *Listening for What Matters: Avoiding Contextual Errors in Health Care*, based on years of research in which they recorded, categorized, and studied over six thousand provider-patient encounters.

Here's a snippet of their impressive body of groundbreaking research: A full 40 percent of the patient encounters they studied had a contextual care issue—an issue that, if not addressed, could cause a medical intervention to fail. And 40 percent of the time in those encounters, the contextual factor was *not* addressed, which means of *all* the patient encounters they studied, 16 percent were not treated appropriately because of a missed contextual issue. That's a one in eight failure rate, which is completely unacceptable and represents a colossal waste of medical treatment. It also represents medical care that could have been redirected if the contextual cues had been picked up.

It gets worse. The type of patient visits that Saul and Alan studied were general medical visits. In a posthospital situation, the impact of contextual factors is much greater. They discovered that contextual errors were the *number one reason* patients ended up with serious failures in the posthospital recovery period. They further found that if contextual factors were not addressed, the chance of a good medical outcome was only 40 percent. Whereas if contextual factors were addressed, that chance goes up to over 70 percent. That's clearly a significant difference in positive outcomes.[80]

One of the important things I learned from Alan and Saul is that contextual care is not the same thing as "caring." In other words, it's not just about having empathy for a patient or a nicer "bedside manner." It has more to do with doing our job as healthcare professionals. It's about understanding those life issues that don't involve illness or disease but still have a profound and immediate impact on one's health outcomes. Saul shared this story to demonstrate that contextual care is largely about two things: (1) taking the time to ask questions and (2) learning how to ask the *right* questions.

> *I had a mentor, a family physician, Simon Oster, who was incredibly influential to me when I was much younger. And he often said, "The best way to show you care is to ask a question." So when someone says, "It's been tough since I've lost my job," you turn to them, and you ask, "How has it been tough since you've lost your job?" To me, that is caring because you're in problem-solving mode. You're actually trying to figure out, okay, what can I do to help this person?*

Over the course of their work, Saul and Alan have developed an approach that operationalizes the steps to asking the right questions. Addressing what they refer to as "contextual gaps" can be accomplished in the following four steps:

---

80   Saul Weiner and Alan Schwartz, *Listening for What Matters: Avoiding Contextual Errors in Health Care* (Oxford: Oxford University Press, 2016).

ADDRESSING GAPS IN CONTEXTUAL CARE

Step 1: Pick up on clues that the patient is experiencing a contextual issue.

Step 2: Ask "fearless questions" that directly address the contextual issue. These questions may feel uncomfortable, but they are necessary to get at the true reality of the situation the patient is encountering.

Step 3: Continue probing until you can identify the root cause of the contextual issue.

Step 4: Create a plan of care to address that issue.

One challenge to Alan and Saul's simple approach is that the current system of care is mostly focused on medical issues, not nonmedical issues. Another part of the problem is time. Contextual care takes time. Still another challenge is payment. For these reasons and others, contextual care is not yet embedded in how we practice medicine. Or to put it bluntly, the healthcare system is conspiring against contextual care. But one company is attempting to change that.

THE LAGUNA HEALTH REVOLUTION

Laguna Health was founded in 2020 by Yoni Shtein and Yael Adam. Both of these entrepreneurs were motivated to create Laguna Health after personal experiences with posthospitalization challenges—Yoni after navigating the complexities of losing a loved one and Yael after multiple surgeries from injuries due to her intense physical activities as a world-class athlete. Having worked together as software engineers at Microsoft, Yael and Yoni established careers in digital health. Laguna leverages their tech backgrounds to radically modernize care management and hospital recovery through tech-enabled, contextual care interventions under the supervision of Laguna's president and chief medical officer, Dr. Alan Spiro.

In 2022 Laguna Health recruited Alan Schwartz and Saul Weiner. The connection point was Dr. Spiro, who had been working with Yael and Yoni, also knew about the contextual care work. Dr. Spiro realized how contextual care protocols could bolster Laguna's efforts to address the nonmedical issues that plague patient recovery after hospital discharge. To that end, Laguna is leveraging AI to systematize contextual care and embed it within state-of-the-art software and digital technology, enabling their care teams to take contextual care to a whole new level.

One specific problem Laguna targets is the high rate and cost of readmission to the hospital when recovery falters or fails. Readmission rates within thirty days of hospital discharge are typically within the 10 to 20 percent range, with rates for some diagnoses being closer to 30 percent.[81] It's a surprisingly high rate of readmissions. The negative impact on patients and their families is profound, especially in terms of morbidity and mortality, stress, and extra medical bills. Health insurance companies experience the added costs. And for hospitals, it presents a quality-of-care problem, a capacity issue, and since 2012 a penalty issue. In 2012 the CMS began to reduce payments to hospitals that had too many patient readmissions within thirty days of their release. Because there was now a penalty attached, healthcare systems began to focus on reducing readmissions. Here's Yoni's take on it:

Hospitals were incentivized to care about this and to improve the recovery journey. But their ability to dramatically influence

---

[81] Audrey Weiss and H. Joanna Jian, "Overview of Clinical Conditions with Frequent and Costly Hospital Readmissions by Payer," Healthcare Cost and Utilization Project, Agency for Healthcare Research and Quality, July 2021, https://hcup-us.ahrq.gov/reports/statbriefs/sb278-Conditions-Frequent-Readmissions-By-Payer-2018.jsp.

that was limited. This is really not their core expertise. What we realized is that we should reframe the conversation from avoiding that thirty-day readmission to looking at the entire recovery journey and any adverse outcomes of that recovery journey.

[An outcome] is certainly adverse if it is preventable. If it's not preventable, then that's just the reality of it. If it is preventable—which over half of the cases turn out to be—it's certainly an adverse event.

What we find interesting about the recovery journey is that it presents this extreme inflection point. A successful recovery journey would essentially entail that patient recovering to a fairly healthy and fairly inexpensive position. Whereas a failed recovery would essentially lead to a spiraling out of control of care outcomes, of life, and of costs.

SYSTEMATIZING CONTEXTUAL CARE

Laguna's objective is to systematize and automate contextual care. To do that, Laguna leverages natural language processing, AI, and a cohort of clinical professionals from disciplines who understand the emotional, relational, and social issues that could hamper full recoveries. Laguna then trains their teams in the four contextual care steps outlined earlier in this chapter.

What I learned from Saul and Alan is that contextual factors fall into two categories: challenges in life circumstances and challenges in behaviors. Within those two categories are defined at least twelve domains that contain contextual issues. Six are based on the patient's healthcare situation, and the other six are more behavioral or interpersonal in nature. The six that are based around care include the following:

1. **Access to care.** This could mean anything from transportation to navigation to scheduling appointments. In other words, how easily can the patient obtain the care they need?

2. **Competing responsibilities.** This takes us back to the story of the woman who needed dialysis but also had to care for an ill child. A patient may have other obligations that keep them from seeking care when they need it.

3. **Social support disruption.** A patient returns home from the hospital, where they have a caregiver, but something happens to that caregiver. Suddenly, the person designated to help in the patient's recovery is out of the picture.

4. **Financial issues.** The patient can't afford the co-payments or medication costs or perhaps is struggling just to buy food or pay rent. Seeking care is put on the back burner because the person is struggling just to get by.

5. **Change in environment.** Perhaps the person has to move. Perhaps there was a loss of power, and they can't store food or medication in the fridge. Whatever the change that has taken place, it impedes the patient from getting proper care.

6. **Change in resources.** The patient has lost a resource that's needed during the recovery phase. Perhaps their car has broken down, and they can't get to the grocery store, let alone to a doctor's office.

The other six domains of contextual issues are behavioral or interpersonal.

7. **Skills, abilities, and knowledge.** The patient could be experiencing cognitive decline, delirium, arthritis, or any other condition that could limit their ability to communicate or physically take care of themselves.

8. **Emotional state.** Anxiety or depression can be major issues and is a big focus of Laguna's efforts. They believe it is probably the biggest contextual factor that is missed by the traditional healthcare system.

9. **Cultural perspectives and spiritual beliefs.** Someone may possess beliefs that interfere with how they interact with the healthcare system.

10. **Attitude toward illness.** People have different ideas about disease and illness. Some try to ignore it. Others think they have a problem when they're perfectly fine. People have different frameworks of understanding that impact how and when they might reach out for help.

11. **Attitude toward the provider and the healthcare system.** Some people distrust the system and those who work within it. This is a big issue in the Black community because the system in the past has victimized them, but many others also have limited trust of practitioners.

12. **Health behavior.** Let's face it, many people have unhealthy lifestyles. They don't exercise enough (or at all), their diet isn't good for them, they routinely miss taking medication, and so on.

CONTEXTUAL CARE CHECKLIST[82]

- Access to care
- Competing responsibilities
- Social support disruption
- Financial issues
- Change in environment
- Change in resources
- Skills, abilities, and knowledge
- Emotional state
- Cultural perspectives and spiritual beliefs
- Attitude toward illness
- Attitude toward the provider and the healthcare system
- Health behavior

How does Laguna keep on top of all these domains? Yoni described their three-pronged approach, which involves (1) a technology-enabled solution with multimodal patient interfaces (telephonic, digital app, and family/caregiver app), (2) a care management platform, and (3) a care engine to orchestrate everything and integrate the clinical and contextual pathways.

First, patients are offered an app that they can download even before their hospitalization. The app connects the patient to the digital software platform. It's the "care journey hub" and can also serve as the tool to prepare patients for surgery or other hospital admissions. Yoni often refers to their approach as a "choose your own journey" because

---

82   Saul Weiner, "Contextualizing Care: An Essential and Measurable Clinical Competency," ScienceDirect, March 2022, https://www.sciencedirect.com/science/article/pii/S0738399121004158.

patients have choices about what part of the technology to use and how to use it. The app is also the channel through which empathetic relationships and trust are built between the patient, their family, and the Laguna care team.

The second prong is called "Harmony." It is a case management tool that is used by Laguna's (or a customer's) care team—a team composed of nurses, pharmacists, and largely behavioral-oriented professionals.

The third prong is what they call the "care engine," which is constantly looking for barriers to care recovery. This prong is Laguna Health's greatest differentiator, and it deserves a bit more explanation. This is where Saul and Alan's two decades of research painstakingly identifying the contextual factors that lead to bad outcomes comes into play. They've programmed the care engine to automatically identify what they call contextual "recovery barriers," to dynamically adjust and personalize the care plan, and when needed, to notify the care management team.

They've also built numerous care protocols into the Harmony case management software so that when the barriers are discovered, there's an evidence-based approach for the care management teams to resolve it. It's the most sophisticated and personalized approach I've encountered when it comes to postprocedure or posthospital recovery. From my perspective, it's the gold standard for contextual care.

Here's an example Yoni shared with me. There was a patient who was at home after a hospital stay. He began to miss taking his medications, and he also wasn't moving about the house as much. The remote app and monitoring devices, as well as questions the app texted to the patient, prompted a contextual coach to call him and do some probing to identify the root cause of these behavior changes. The outcome? This man had a urinary tract infection that was causing him to become exhausted and confused, therefore leading him to miss his medications and also to be more bedbound at home. Armed with that knowledge, Laguna was able to get him treated with antibiotics at home and back on the road to recovery.

That was a relatively simple fix but also a relatively simple miss had it not been picked up by the combination of technology and care teams at Laguna. A more complex example of contextual care is that of a patient in cardiac rehab, which typically begins six weeks after a discharge. Even at the best health systems in the country, the engagement rate of cardiac rehab is in the single-digit range. In other words, less than 10 percent of the patients who would benefit from cardiac rehab actually do it. Laguna has the ability to monitor patients' entire recovery journey and make sure they begin and stay engaged in lifesaving programs such as cardiac rehab.

Laguna has been putting their approach to the test. In 2021 they launched a trial with Northshore University Health System to test their model. In 2023 they released the results of the trial showing a nearly 50 percent decrease in total readmission costs.[83] As they say, the proof is in the pudding, and that's some pretty impressive pudding.

I believe that integrating contextual care into everyday patient encounters may be one of the most important reframes to occur in healthcare—with tremendous benefit for patients, providers, and payers. It's clear this is a huge gap in American healthcare delivery today, and it's going to take 'beyond the walls' ventures such as Laguna to assist us in filling the hole. In the next chapter, we're going to see an example of another such venture—a national effort to bring Whole Health to one of the most deserving segments of American citizens, our veterans.

---

83   Iva Minga et al., "A Personalized Approach to the Post-Acute Hospitalization Recovery Journey; a Novel Intervention for Improving Patient Experience and Reducing Cost," *Journal of the American College of Cardiology* 81, no, 8_Supplement (March 2023): 531, https://doi.org/10.1016/S0735-1097(23)00975-0.

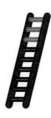

CHAPTER 6
WHOLE-PERSON HEALTH

We're currently not tapping into one of the most powerful sources of health, which is really a person's ability to make changes in their life, to move forward in their life, towards what's important to them and to really address what's keeping them from having a whole and healthy life.
—Dr. Ben Kligler, MD, MPH, Veterans Health Administration

The entrepreneurs we've profiled in part II focus on providing care that addresses all aspects of a patient's life. But they've done more than just focus on it; they've operationalized it by integrating it as a core part of clinical care delivery. In this chapter, we're going to discover a national 'beyond the walls' movement that is currently situated *within* the walls of the Veteran Health Affairs (VHA) system. They've managed to make Whole Health their foundational form of care.

The Whole Health movement attempts to understand people's needs and priorities—not just medical needs but also *human* needs such as emotional, relational, and spiritual needs—and the sense of purpose and meaning in their lives. The intent is to directly address the worsening health outcomes of individuals as well as of the American public. Once again, our clinically constrained approach is insufficient. We need, as I learned from Dr. Ben Kligler, to "widen the aperture." Whole Health, as you'll discover in the following pages, is an idea whose time has come. Quite frankly, it's come in the nick of time.

WHAT IS WHOLE HEALTH?

The Whole Health movement is a river fed by many streams, and it's been gaining great momentum over the past couple of decades. From my reading, a single unified definition has yet to be codified, but someone who has a great handle on the concept is Dr. Ben Kligler.

Dr. Benjamin Kligler is a board-certified family physician. He's a clinician, an educator, and a researcher and has been a leader in the field of complementary and integrative medicine for over twenty-five years. In May 2016 he was named the national director of the Integrative Health Coordinating Center in the Office of Patient Centered Care and Cultural Transformation at the Veterans Administration, as well as the director of Education and Research for Whole Health. In May 2020 he was named executive director of that same office.

To Ben, Whole Health is an opportunity, as he puts it, "to look at the whole person and to ask the question of what matters to them, to change the conversation. We're still going to provide the best medical care but do it in the context of really understanding a patient much better as a person and really engaging them and what's important to them."

What Ben is tapping into is the desire for medical care that goes beyond the transactional, that goes beyond treating disease and illness, while still acknowledging that those are critically important and necessary. Whole Health recognizes that people's health and health-care are a part of something much bigger—their lives. Within the Whole Health framework, medical providers need to understand not just what's the matter with us but also what matters *to* us.

While Whole Health is, by definition, highly inclusive, it isn't defined by any one of its component modalities, such as lifestyle medicine, integrative

> Medical providers need to understand not just what's the matter with us but also what matters to us.

medicine, or even the SDOH. It isn't an alternative medicine of any sort. When Ben describes Whole Health as "widening the aperture" of care delivery, he's talking about moving beyond the "find it and fix it" framework to a purpose-driven framework.

WHOLE HEALTH AND PRIORITIZING PURPOSE

In order to rapidly scale the Whole Health movement within the VHA, Ben and his colleagues distilled its essence to the following two foundational questions:

TWO ESSENTIAL WHOLE HEALTH QUESTIONS

1. What is most important to you, in your life, right now?
2. What is the thing that you would be willing and able to do today or tomorrow to move closer to that?

Just let those two questions sink in. Imagine what it would feel like if your PCP asked them as a standing part of your visit.

In the VHA's Whole Health program, providers and their teams can begin to gain some perspective into what matters to the patient (their priorities and purpose) and how to assist and empower them to live the life they want to live. One remarkable thing is that not only are these questions becoming a standard part of patient care, but the responses are also being recorded in the electronic medical record as a way to ensure that the entire care team is aware and continuously supporting the patient's purpose.

Why is this focus on purpose so important? I was surprised to learn that having a sense of purpose is associated with health and longevity. Ben shared that individuals with a low sense of purpose are two and a half times more likely to die than those with a high sense of purpose. His stats are backed by a body of research showing that those who have a strong life purpose actually live longer. In one cohort study of 6,985 adults,[84] results indicated that possessing a stronger purpose in life was associated with a significant decrease in mortality. Another fourteen-year study had similar findings and concluded that "having a purpose in life appears to widely buffer against mortality risk across the adult years."[85]

A more anecdotal but incredibly powerful confirmation of this link between life and purpose can be found in *Man's Search for Meaning*, written by psychiatrist Viktor Frankl. In 1991 the Library of Congress cited it as one of the ten most meaningful books in the United States. During WWII, Dr. Frankl was held captive in several

---

84   Aliya Alimujiang et al., "Association between Life Purpose and Mortality among US Adults Older Than 50 Years," *JAMA Network Open* 2, no. 5 (May 24, 2019): e194270, https://doi.org/10.1001/jamanetworkopen.2019.4270.

85   Patrick L. Hill and Nicholas A. Turiano, "Purpose in Life as a Predictor of Mortality across Adulthood," *Psychological Science* 25, no. 7 (July 2014):1482–6, https://doi.org/10.1177/0956797614531799.

Nazi concentration camps, including the infamous Auschwitz death camp. He observed that camp occupants who felt they had the most to live for were more likely to survive the brutal conditions than those who could not find an overarching purpose for their lives. Those who survived were not the strongest, the smartest, or the cleverest. The ones who survived were those who could find and maintain a sense of purpose, even under those harshest of inhumane conditions. Purpose, as it turns out, is not just a way to live a more meaningful life; it's also a way to live a longer life.

WHOLE HEALTH AND A FOCUS ON RELATIONSHIPS

Similar to the focus on life purpose, the Whole Health approach also emphasizes and evaluates relationships, not just as a motivator for healthful behaviors but also as a core determinant of health outcomes and longevity. The role of relationship quality in health and longevity is no longer a matter of opinion or hypotheses but is made evident in a thoroughly researched set of scientific findings. Among other studies, what ranks as the longest and largest study in this area is the Harvard Study of Adult Development, also referred to as "the happiness study." This ongoing study began in 1938 and closely followed over 700 male participants from adolescence to the end of their lives. In the 1970s the study was broadened to include the wives of the study participants, and in the 2000s it was expanded to include over 1,300 of their sons and daughters. My initial impression of the study was that it only included white male Harvard undergrads, but I was completely incorrect in this assumption. The study also drew in individuals from poor immigrant families all over the Boston area. A recent book, *The Good Life*[86]—coauthored by Dr. Robert Waldinger, a professor of psychiatry at the Harvard Medical School and the current lead of the Harvard Study of Adult Development, and Marc Schulz, a professor of psychology and director of data science at Bryn Mawr College—points out the following five key insights on the association of relationships to health, happiness, and longevity:

1. Good relationships keep us happier and healthier, and their absence diminishes our health and well-being. Lonely people live shorter lives, and chronic loneliness increases a person's odds of death, in any given year, by 26 percent.

2. Relationships require active maintenance. Not addressing relationships as a determinant of health and longevity could be compared to not addressing high blood pressure or cigarette smoking. They should be as pertinent an item on a patient's problem list as any other.

3. Relationships of all kinds matter—family, friends, coworkers, and even casual relationships—but they do come with challenges that need to be addressed. Many, if not most people, struggle with challenging aspects of relationships, and learning how to navigate these challenges is critical.

4. Maintaining and nurturing relationships requires time, and that requires intention and commitment. Relationships require a plan of action.

5. It's never too late to improve relationships and connectivity with others and experience a positive impact on one's health outcomes.

---

86 Robert Waldinger and Marc Schulz, *The Good Life: Lessons from the World's Longest Scientific Study of Happiness* (New York: Simon & Schuster, 2023).

The overarching takeaway point here is that the VA's Whole Health approach has elevated the focus on relationships to a core determinant of health and an integral component of clinical care delivery. This is a new and important contribution to clinical medicine and healthcare delivery, and it should be duly noted.

WHOLE HEALTH ENCOMPASSES OTHER DETERMINANTS OF HEALTH

Whole Health is a collaborative approach that leverages an individual's sense of purpose, autonomy, and capabilities as drivers of engagement and of healthcare delivery. As such, it's not an alternative, a complementary, or an ancillary approach. Ben and his colleagues at the VHA believe that it is the foundation of a successful healthcare system. As Ben put it, "We are creating an actual delivery system built on Whole Health. It is core, critical, and necessary if we are to achieve the desired goals."

But Whole Health is not solely focused at the level of the individual patient. It also smartly expands the aperture by adopting a population health and public health mindset and addressing issues such as medication adherence, clinical outcomes of care, and cost-effectiveness of care. It takes into account the SDOH, cultural sensitivities, and disparities of care, including issues of implicit bias and racism. Years of research demonstrate that the nonclinical determinants of health have a much bigger impact on health outcomes than the clinical factors. For example, a study from the University of Wisconsin Population Health Institute found that only 20 percent of healthcare outcomes result from clinical care. Health behaviors accounted for 30 percent of the impact, physical environment accounted for 10 percent of the impact, and social and environmental factors accounted for 40 percent of the impact on health outcomes.[87]

Recognizing this body of research, the only rational, practical, and ethical thing to do is to resource the Whole Health approach, integrate it into daily healthcare delivery, and spread it. That is exactly what the VHA is doing—spreading it to every VA hospital and clinic across the nation. It's a credit to the courageous 'beyond the walls' leadership at the VHA. As Ben shared with me, "What's great about our situation in the VA is we've had really forward-looking leaders in our health system who've been willing to say 'Okay, this may not be the way mainstream healthcare looks at its job, but we're going to start looking at it this way.' Our Whole Health System of Care is really much bigger than any particular program or even model of care because it's really about a paradigm shift and a transformation in how we think about our job."

The VHA has prioritized Whole Health because they see it as the key to delivering optimal healthcare outcomes in the most humanistic way possible. Here, Ben describes why the VHA has made Whole Health a top priority:

> Not that we want to give up our success with high-tech medicine and with some of the really amazing disease-oriented inter-ventions we've developed. But we've just hit a wall, and there are things we can't address with those approaches. People are feeling isolated and stuck. That's why I think Whole Health is a must-have. And I think there's a compelling argument for doing Whole Health in the VA because of the many different challenges that veterans face, challenges that go beyond just managing

---

87   "County Health Rankings Model," County Health Rankings & Roadmaps, University of Wisconsin Population Health Institute, 2023, https://www.countyhealthrankings.org/explore-health-rankings/county-health-rankings-model.

their diabetes or their hypertension or whatever other medical problem they have.

THE THREE PARTS OF THE WHOLE HEALTH SYSTEM

The first part of the VHA's Whole Health System is called the *Pathway*, and it has three components: an assessment, a selection of what to work on, and an action plan. The assessment is a Personal Health Inventory (PHI), which addresses what's most important to a person right now and what that person wants to work on. It also identifies areas of strength as well as areas where some assistance might be needed. The PHI is placed in the electronic medical record to assure that Whole Health becomes an integral part of that person's care. According to Ben, once the PHI is completed, it's a "choose your own adventure" scenario because patients custom build their own programs. This customization is available through the VHA's "Wheel of Health," which offers eight different domains of self-care to explore. These domains include nutrition, physical activity, mindfulness, relationships, personal development, spiritual health, recharging, and physical and emotional surroundings. You can view the actual Wheel of Health on the program website.[88] Once an individual has decided on a few areas they'd like to focus on, the next step is setting personalized goals. The goal setting can be done on their own or with their clinical team, a health coach, a designated Whole Health partner, or a peer-to-peer counselor. The goals are designed to be specific, measurable, and achievable. A goal might be to walk thirty minutes a day on Mondays, Wednesdays, and Fridays for the next three weeks.

---

88 "Whole Health," US Department of Veterans Affairs, accessed March 23, 2023, https://www.va.gov/wholehealth/.

The second part of the Whole Health system is called the *Well-Being Program*. It includes classes in nutrition, tai chi, yoga, meditation, and health coaching. It also includes access to complementary therapies such as acupuncture, biofeedback, and clinical hypnosis—all of which are covered by the veterans' medical benefits.

The third component is *Whole Health Clinical Care*—engaging in Whole Health during regular medical visits with a primary care team or specialists. Two points Ben makes about Whole Health Clinical Care are that it doesn't really take more time during clinical visits, and the results more than justify the small additional effort.

Veterans can engage with the Whole Health program through any and all of these pathways, either with their provider and care team, or through the peer-to-peer program, or with specially trained Whole Health experts (Whole Health Partners) that are being deployed at every veteran medical center. The VHA has a growing network of veterans who are trained as facilitators to have these conversations with their fellow veterans. These peer-to-peer interactions could be one-on-one or in a group setting and can also take place virtually.

The VHA's approach to Whole Health is being scaled and spread nationally to over 140 medical centers plus hundreds of ambulatory care sites. The sophisticated operation is being resourced appropriately and includes the following:

- Training programs of different lengths and depths for providers and staff taught by a national faculty that travels throughout the country

- The placement of on-site faculty and experts at medical centers

- The development of peer coaches and health coaches

- Having providers and staff themselves experience the Whole Health approach to help them make the shift from the "What's the matter with you?" to the "What matters to you?" mindset

VALIDATION OF WHOLE HEALTH

Of course, the big question is, does Whole Health deliver on its promise? Here's how Ben describes some of their early observations:

We've seen that veterans with lower back pain who used Whole Health ended up requiring a significantly lower number of invasive spine procedures over the subsequent eighteen months. We looked at the rates of epidural injections, low back surgeries, and implanted stimulator devices in veterans who used Whole Health versus veterans who didn't and found between a 20 percent and 40 percent decrease in the number of procedures required, once people were engaged in Whole Health.

On a quantitative level, we've been doing some pretty rigorous analyses of outcomes at our eighteen flagship sites. Some of the most impressive things we found are that the veterans who were using Whole Health, compared to the veterans who didn't, had a 38 percent drop over the course of a year in their average opioid dose. Basically, the veterans who chose Whole Health were able to reduce their dosing by three and a half times the degree of people who didn't. It's an observational study, but at the same time, that's a very meaningful outcome.

We also have data showing that when employees are more engaged with Whole Health at their facility, they have lower burnout, they have lower turnover intent, and they score higher on what they call the "Best Places to Work" scale. We have some preliminary data that shows that creating this as part of the environment that people work in has really substantial benefits for the staff as well.

It's clear that the VHA is seeing positive qualitative and quantitative outcomes emerging from its Whole Health mandate. A couple of other outcomes are related to appropriately reduced costs of care.[89] Patients who used the Whole Health program only saw an increase in outpatient pharmacy costs for mental health conditions of 3.5 percent, compared to a 12.5 percent increase in costs for those patients who did not use the program. And, patients who used the Whole Health program only saw an increase in outpatient pharmacy costs for chronic conditions of 4.3 percent, compared to a 15.8 percent increase in costs for those patients who did not use the program.

Along these same lines, another expert I've had the opportunity to interview is Connor D. Drake, PhD, a faculty member of the Duke University School of Medicine and a research scientist at the Veterans Health Administration. Connor's research is focused on Whole Health and "whole person" care models. He also cofounded ZealCare, a company whose mission is to manage complex chronic diseases through tech-enabled engagement with patients and their caregivers. To Connor and his colleagues, the evidence is clear: care models with a Whole Health orientation can improve both patient experience and clinical outcomes, particularly for those people who are at higher risk for cardiometabolic diseases such as diabetes, heart attacks, and strokes. It works, in part, through promoting sustainable lifestyle changes, improving medication adherence, increasing the use of preventive primary care, and helping patients avoid preventable ED visits and hospitalizations. The net result is better outcomes and the ability to achieve cost savings for patients who are already driving high costs or those who are predicted to do so. In one study Connor cited,

---

89 "Whole System of Care Evaluation: A Progress Report on Outcomes of the WHS Pilot at 18 Flagship Sites," Infographic, US Department of Veterans Affairs, February 18, 2020, https://www.va.gov/WHOLEHEALTH/docs/WH-Evaluation-One-Sheet-infographics-06082020-508.pdf.

researchers observed a cost savings of $7,000 to $9,000 up through eighteen months after program completion.[90]

THE MOST COMPELLING VALIDATION OF WHOLE HEALTH

At present the most compelling validation and endorsement for the Whole Health movement may come not from a research study but from a 406-page report put out by the National Academies of Science, Engineering, and Medicine in early 2023.[91] The committee authoring this report studied the VA's Whole Health system and concluded that it could benefit all people across the country, not just veterans. As Dr. Alex Krist, committee cochair, stated, "We believe it is possible for Whole Health approaches to be expanded to the rest of the US health-care system, with enormous potential benefits for all." The study adds that the VA and HHS should collaborate to create a Whole Health Innovation Center modeled after CMS's Innovation Center and the federal Cancer Moonshot initiative.

Another validation of the Whole Health movement comes from a 2023 report published by the US surgeon general Dr. Vivek Murthy. In this detailed report, he states, "We need a shift in perspective to an upstream 'whole-person health' approach aimed at providing the tools and resources that individuals and communities need to face today's challenges, before they develop downstream consequences." He concluded, "The responses to the central question asked in whole-person health, 'What matters to you?' should inform public health

---

90   George L. Jackson et al., "Benefits of Participation in Diabetes Group Visits after Trial Completion," *JAMA Internal Medicine* 173, no. 7 (2013): 590–592, https://doi.org/10.1001/jamainternmed.2013.2803.

91   National Academies of Sciences, Engineering, and Medicine, *Achieving Whole Health: A New Approach for Veterans and the Nation* (Washington, DC: The National Academies Press, 2023), https://doi.org/10.17226/26854.

policy and practice at the individual, family, and community levels.… 'What matters' … must inspire us to invest in resources, align leadership, shift structures, and direct systems and services to meet these fundamental needs."[92] This is a clear call from the surgeon general to reframe our public health policies and approaches within the context of Whole Health. It's an endorsement at the highest level.

And there is one more validation: the financial and economic imperative for spreading Whole Health throughout the American population. Healthcare spending in the United States is approximately $3.8 trillion (nearly 18 percent of the US GDP) and projected to reach nearly $6.2 trillion by 2028 and $11.8 trillion by 2040. A team of actuaries at Deloitte recently calculated that the US healthcare system could reduce that 2040 cost trajectory to $8.3 trillion by adopting "well-being" as a mainstay of care. They dubbed the potential $3.5 trillion savings a "well-being dividend."[93] That's a return on investment that could be accrued if we put the tools, systems, and protocols in place that would enable consumers to take a more active role in their health and well-being.

The team at Deloitte defined "well-being" as "wholistic (versus holistic), where the health of the whole individual is considered. This includes physical and mental health as well as spiritual, social, emotional, equitable, and even financial health." In this report, the authors made two more predictions about the future. First, they predict a seismic shift in the way that healthcare dollars will be spent. In 2019 approximately 80 percent of all healthcare spending went to clinical care and treatment or what some have termed "sick care." They believe that by 2040, 60 percent of all spending will go toward

92   Vivek Murthy, "The Time Is Now for a Whole-Person Health Approach to Public Health," *Public Health Reports* (February 2023), https://doi.org/10.1177/00333549231154583.

93   Kulleni Gebreyes et al., "Breaking the Cost Curve: Deloitte Predicts Health Spending as a Percentage of GDP Will Decelerate over the Next 20 Years," *Deloitte Insights*, February 9, 2021, https://www2.deloitte.com/us/en/insights/industry/health-care/future-health-care-spending.html.

improving health and well-being. Second, they predict a "new health economy, different from today's business models, will drive 85 percent of all revenue." New business models will focus on well-being and care enablement, as well as care delivery data and platforms. We'll dive into the platform revolution in chapter 7, but the inescapable point here is that the mounting clinical, public health, and economic evidence is compelling us to adopt a Whole Health movement as the foundation of American healthcare.

CHALLENGES TO WHOLE HEALTH IMPLEMENTATION

Despite the growing documentation that demonstrates the effectiveness of the Whole Health approach, the movement still faces some formidable challenges, especially if it is to be adopted outside of the VHA.

First, not everyone agrees on what Whole Health *is*. This may change, now that the VA has scaled and is integrating a specific program within its healthcare system. The administration has a clear method and approach and is rigorously studying the outcomes.

Second, there are numerous other issues, such as affordability and access, battling for priority. So it may be difficult for systems outside of the VHA to see where Whole Health fits into their current priorities. I would argue, however, that the solution won't be found in trying to make the current system more efficient but in adopting the humanistic 'beyond the walls' movements described here in part II.

Perhaps the biggest obstacle to Whole Health implementation outside of the VHA is finding a viable payment model. Currently, our healthcare system relies on an FFS model. For Whole Health to succeed, there will need to be a transition to a value-based model like what we see in the VHA. Put very simply, the VHA receives a set amount of money for each veteran enrolled in its care and decides how best to spend that money to optimize health. Since most veterans remain in the system for years, the investment is a worthwhile one. This may be one of the primary reasons why the VHA is leading the Whole Health movement. And it may be one of the primary reasons why hospital-based healthcare systems and other entrenched legacy stakeholders across the country might resist it.

A YEARNING FOR WHOLE HEALTH

All of the innovations we've discussed so far in this book are rooted in an effort to take healthcare beyond the walls and make it a part of people's everyday lives in a proactive and empathic way.

I believe that the VHA has hit upon a core and unmet consumer desire for a different type of dialogue, different interactions, and different relationships in the delivery of healthcare. Underneath all of the interviews I've conducted over the past few years—whether the discussions were about value-based payment models, innovative care models, advanced analytics, digital health, or consumer experience— is a yearning among patients to be listened to and understood as a whole person. That yearning to have our healthcare be guided by the meaning and context of our lives and to be recognized and respected as autonomous beings is a yearning to live the best lives we can.

I believe that healthcare providers desire this as much as their patients, as reflected in the burgeoning literature on the "moral injury" that doctors, nurses, and other providers are experiencing.[94] In 2022 a study published in *Mayo Clinic Proceedings* reported that 63 percent of physicians surveyed were experiencing at least one symptom of burnout. This is compared with 44 percent in 2017 and 38 percent in early 2020.

---

94   Eric Reinhart, "Doctors Aren't Burned Out from Overwork. We're Demoralized by Our Health System," *New York Times*, February 5, 2023.

The pandemic no doubt contributed to the increase, but there seems to be more to it. Dr. Tait Shanafelt, an oncologist at Stanford who helped write a 312-page report on physician burnout for the National Academy of Medicine, said, "Evidence suggested that many doctors' dissatisfaction with their work could be caused by an incongruence between what they cared about and what they were incentivized to do by the health care system."[95] Dr. Victor Dzau, president of the National Academy of Medicine, shares this perspective and sees the Whole Health approach as helping to resolve workforce issues: "Whole health is an approach that holds great potential for addressing major challenges in health care workforce well-being that have only intensified in recent years."[96]

Dr. Ben Kligler and his colleagues at the VHA provide an approach to address the fundamental problem that is preventing providers from delivering the type of relational care they desire. Whole Health is a reframe that will enable us to experience a more humanistic approach to healthcare delivery in America. It may be the largest and most significant humanistic shift occurring right now in the American healthcare system. In the next chapter, which kicks off the final section of this book, we're going to explore how tech-enabled platforms can scale humanistic healthcare connectivity beyond what was possible or even thinkable before now.

> Whole Health is an approach that holds great potential for addressing major challenges in health care workforce well-being that have only intensified in recent years.

---

95 Oliver Whang, "Physician Burnout Has Reached Distressing Levels, New Research Finds," *New York Times,* September 29, 2022, https://www.nytimes.com/2022/09/29/health/doctor-burnout-pandemic.html.

96 National Academies of Sciences, Engineering, and Medicine, "U.S. Should Scale and Spread Whole Health Care through VA and HHS Leadership, Create Federal Center for Whole Health Innovation, Says New Report," Washington, DC, February 15, 2023.

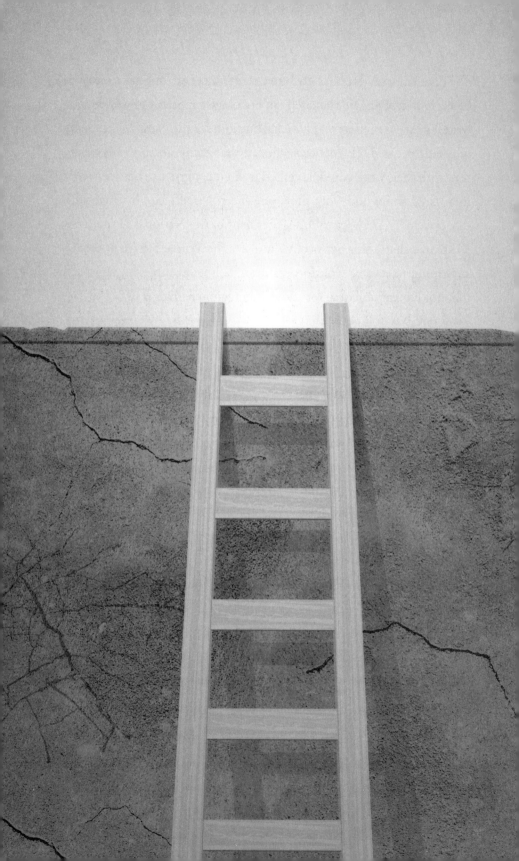

PART III

MARKET DISRUPTORS

We've had a proliferation of technology solutions, many of them are standalone point solutions. But platforms are coming together to change all that, bringing a more coherent experience, a coherent technical architecture, and a new set of business models and better outcomes. That's happening today. We're at the early stages, but this is something already underway.

–Sara Vaezy, chief digital and strategy officer, Providence Health

IN PART I WE REVIEWED the 'beyond the walls' movement in American healthcare in its literal meaning—that is, the transposition of healthcare beyond the physical walls of clinics, emergency rooms, and hospitals. In part II we introduced the humanistic healthcare movements that illustrate the conceptual 'beyond the walls' reformation in American healthcare. In this third and final part of our exploration, we will consider the 'beyond the walls' movement from a systemic perspective.

In chapter 7 we will discover the platform revolution that has radically transformed numerous other industries and is just now beginning to have similar impacts on healthcare delivery. In chapter 8 we will discuss the megabrands that have already entered the healthcare industry and are acting as "titans of disruption." These influencers include the largest online and brick-and-mortar retailers, such as Amazon and Walmart; the largest retail pharmacy chains, such as CVS and Walgreens; and the largest healthcare insurance companies, such as UnitedHealth Group and Humana. In chapter 9, we balance out the picture by describing a 'beyond the walls' strategy that legacy hospital-based healthcare systems are taking—partnerships.

Regarding the use of the word *disruption*, as well as *disruptors* and *disruptive*, you may have noticed that these three words are missing from most of the pages leading up to this section. I've intentionally minimized the use of that verbiage, up until now, for a reason. Those words or, more accurately, the way they are used can be misleading. When used by legacy stakeholders, they can conceal a status quo mindset and an anchoring bias toward keeping things the same. The connotation being that disruption is bad, and therefore, that disruptors are bad. When used by new entrants or other external stakeholders, disruption is often lauded for the harm it's causing the legacy stakeholders. Either form of misguided usage, whether by legacy stakeholders or new entrants, is self-serving and misses the point. The point isn't about disruption. It's about advancement. While disruption may be a secondary consequence, the primary purpose of these and other disruptors is, or

> The point isn't about disruption. It's about advancement.

should be, to advance the cause. I once read that Jeff Bezos chided his teams to *not* concern themselves with competitors but instead focus their attention, time, and energy on customers. He understood the prime directive, which is to create value for consumers—a lesson that all of us in healthcare would be wise to heed.

So here's a thought experiment. Instead of labeling transformative change "disruption," could we label it "advancement"? And could we shift from labeling innovators as "disruptors" to describing them as advancers, whether they be new entrants or legacy stakeholders who are advancing healthcare delivery? I have discussed this "advancement" reframe with a number of healthcare executives and found that it's going to take a little bit of time for it to catch on. In the meantime, in order to maintain congruence and readability, I'll use the widely accepted notion of transformative individuals and organizations being labeled as "disruptors." Just keep in mind that what they're disrupting is a system that is not meeting the needs of the American public, a system that is in crisis on multiple fronts, and a system that is unsustainable. That said, there may be a virtuous consequence of using the "disruption" verbiage. It can be used by leaders as a catalyst to motivate change and advancement.

Another new perspective to broaden our understanding of disruption comes from W. Chan Kim and Renee Mauborgne, authors of the best-selling book Blue Ocean Strategy. In a recent Harvard Business Review article, they write, "For the past 20 years 'disruption' has been a battle cry in business. Not surprisingly, many have come to see it as a near-synonym for innovation. But the obsession with disruption obscures an important truth: Market-creating innovation isn't always disruptive."[97]

---

97   W. Chan Kim and Renee Mauborgne, "Innovation Doesn't Have to Be Disruptive," *Harvard Business Review*, May/June 2023.

In their new book, *Beyond Disruption*, the authors provide numerous business examples of a spectrum of disruption—from "creative disruption" to what they term "non-disruptive creation." Their examples of non-disruptiive creation include e-sports, environmental consulting, the cruise industry, micro-financing, and life coaching. They also include Square (now Block) which was cofounded by Jim McKelvey, who inspired the title of this book. Making sure not to minimize the extent or tremendous impact of disruptive innovation, their point is that business model innovation can create new opportunities, new growth, and new value—advancement—"without displacing any existing markets, players, or jobs".[98]

These two reframes—of advancement and non-disruptive transformation—are woven throughout the examples in this book. I believe they are necessary leadership mindsets if we are to advance new and emerging business models, partnerships, and collaborations that will lead us toward a better future.

---

98 Ibid.

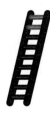

CHAPTER 7

THE BURNING PLATFORM

The way that I think about a platform in the context of healthcare is when you're caring for a patient, there's a need for many different specific expertise. How do you connect the care teams and access the best-in-class support services across all of the types of things that patients may need and make that seem frictionless?
—Caitlin Donovan, global head, Uber Health

I n this chapter we're going to make a seemingly abrupt transition—from contextual and whole-person health to transactional platforms. But as I hope you'll come to appreciate, just like the digital health revolution, these transactional platforms have the potential to greatly enhance the humanistic transformation of healthcare delivery.

An online platform can be a real game changer, the kind that can completely reinvent an existing business sector and revolutionize how products and services are delivered. I'm sure that many of you have purchased items from Amazon. Regular customers know the breadth and depth of what this site offers in terms of selection, convenience, price and product comparisons, fast shipping, and even the ability to stream movies and TV shows. That's the power of a platform at work. Amazon is one of the biggest and most elaborate platforms in existence, and its impact is undeniable. Think about how this retail paradigm has decimated shopping malls from coast to coast. After all, why should you get in your car or onto a bus, navigate traffic and then the crowds, only to confront the possibility that the store you've visited might not even have the product you want? With Amazon, it's all there, literally at your fingertips. It's no wonder that Amazon's marketplace sales have grown from 3 percent of gross merchandise value in 2000 to 62 percent in 2020.[99]

Uber is another excellent example of a disruptive platform. Like Amazon, Uber is a two-sided marketplace that brings buying consumers together with sellers of a service. Like Amazon, Uber started in one focused area—transportation—and now through Uber Eats, it delivers restaurant food and groceries, provides courier services, and more. You can use the Uber app to schedule a ride on-demand, track and speak to your driver before they arrive, and handle payment all through your phone. And you have options, from less expensive cars to larger and more luxurious vehicles. Why call or wait for a taxi when you can easily schedule a ride with Uber? Similar to Amazon's platform, Uber has witnessed significant growth. In 2016 fewer than 25 million people used Uber each quarter. Just seven years later, that number has grown to over 125 million. Uber and its rival, Lyft, have come to dominate taxi utilization. For example, in New York, Uber

99 "Amazon Small Business Empowerment Report," Amazon, 2021, https://assets.abou-tamazon.com/9b/84/05cb2fc14da18e4574a5132f675a/amazon-smb-report-2021.pdf.

completes 435,000 rides a day compared with 105,000 for yellow taxi rides.[100, 101]

Robust platforms profoundly transform the traditional consumer experience by providing more options, more accessibility, and a more efficient delivery of goods and services. That's why, as of March 2023, four out of five of the most valuable companies in the world (by market cap) are powered by platforms.[102]

Now imagine a *healthcare* platform with that kind of transformative power.

> Four out of five of the most valuable companies in the world (by market cap) are powered by platforms.

CURATING VERSUS CREATING

You'll note this chapter is titled "The *Burning* Platform." That term comes from an infamous memo sent by the CEO of Nokia back in 2011, when he compared their company's position to a story about a worker stranded on an oil rig in the middle of the North Sea. The oil rig worker had woken up to an explosion and discovered that the platform he was standing on was on fire. His only option was to make a thirty-meter (nearly one hundred foot) jump into the freezing ocean waters below. He jumped. At the time Nokia was on the ropes because of the iPhone's sudden and overwhelming popularity; Nokia was desperate to find a way to survive. The CEO's call to action was, unfortunately, too late.

100 "Uber Technologies Inc Statistics & Facts," WallStreetZen, accessed March 24, 2023, https://www.wallstreetzen.com/stocks/us/nyse/uber/statistics.

101 Brian Dean, "Uber Statistics 2022: How Many People Ride with Uber?" Backlinko, March 23, 2023, https://backlinko.com/uber-users.

102 "Largest Companies by Market Cap," CompaniesMarketCap.com, https://compa-niesmarketcap.com/.

Today the healthcare industry is standing on a burning platform, and it needs to jump. Why should it be easier to buy just about anything on Amazon and get it delivered for free within two days than to schedule an appointment with your doctor or get the results of your MRI or find a competitive price on your prescription?

These are questions that Dr. Randy Williams and Vince Kuraitis have been asking for years. These two healthcare veterans are literally writing the book on what a healthcare platform business model could and should be. Randy is an experienced physician and healthcare executive. He is currently the managing director of Digital Care Advisors, a healthcare consulting firm, and has advised both the George W. Bush and the Barack Obama administrations on issues related to healthcare reform. Vince is a principal and founder of Better Health Technologies, which helps develop strategic partnerships and business models with a unique focus on platform strategies. He has vast experience in the industry, serving as president of Health Choice, a medical call center, and as VP of Corporate Development and Specialty Operations at Saint Alphonsus Regional Medical Center.

I had an opportunity to meet this duo and hear them speak at a 2022 MIT symposium on platforms. When I interviewed them on my podcast, I realized how the right platform could bring more accessibility, affordability, and equity to healthcare delivery, as well as create fresh approaches to almost all of the challenges we've named in this book. It's important to recognize that platforms are not a future phenomenon. They've been evolving for some time. In fact, the presentation I attended was actually part of the 10th Annual Platform Symposium at MIT. Vince explains the early efforts and why they stalled.

My journey down the platform rabbit hole actually began in 2007, and it happened when Randy, who was then a client, asked me a question. "I see these new powerful business models—Amazon, Google, Facebook. Is there anything here for health-care?" And that was the beginning. I began writing a book on this topic in 2013 but concluded I was about a decade too early. But now, at this point, there are over forty books written on platforms and platform strategy applied to general industry. We're writing the one that's going to be specific for healthcare.

Randy picks up the story from there.

We started to learn about the power of connections, the power of collaborations, the power of shared learning across broad geographies, and what that pointed to was an opportunity to think more creatively about how we could use those connections to drive value, both for patients as well as for provider organizations. And that led us down this path of thinking about something called "network effects" and the power of platforms to execute network effect opportunities.

Platforms offer a huge opportunity for connecting and coordinating all the disparate, fragmented strands of healthcare delivery. The basic difference between platforms and traditional business processes boils down to their sphere of influence on basic business model design. Traditional businesses follow a linear process. There's a straight pipeline from supply chain and manufacturing to selling. In contrast, a platform is all about making connections between producers and users, so in its simplest form, it is a triangle with the platform itself serving as the third point.

TRADITIONAL PLATFORM STRUCTURE
(Producers and Consumers Are outside the Platform)

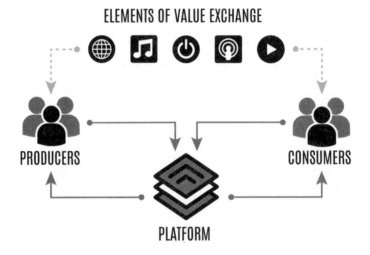

Vince explains the triangle model as follows:[103]

If you think of a health system as a pipeline or a traditional business, it's about gathering raw components, pharmaceuticals, medical devices of various types; bringing in specialized labor and clinicians; and putting that all together along with applying some sort of a through line. Hopefully, you get a healthy patient at the end.

But you could also conceptualize at least parts of a health system through a platform model. And one way to do that is to think of a platform as, again, making connections. You've got patients out there with unique needs, and you've got clinicians in the community that have unique capabilities. How do you best match the patient and the clinician?

---

103   2016 Parker & Van Alstyne, with Choudary—licensed under Creative Commons Attribution-ShareAlike 4.0 International (CC BY-SA 4.0).

What Vince and Randy are getting at is this: a platform is more about curating and aggregating products and services than producing them. Amazon, Airbnb, and other platforms present consumers with products the platform doesn't actually manufacture in order to match consumers with vendors that provide the best fit for their specific needs. In fact, Amazon's e-commerce marketplace sells more stuff from third-party vendors than from Amazon itself. This speaks both to the power of platforms and the counterintuitive value of allowing competitors onto a platform.

> A platform is more about curating and aggregating products and services than producing them.

Let's demonstrate this with two real-life examples. First, consider how Vince describes Airbnb:

> *Airbnb has started to completely disrupt the traditional brick-and-mortar business of the hospitality industry and hotels by operating as a classic platform business. What it's doing—instead of building and assembling hotel space and then selling that to customers like you and me—is actually allowing outsiders to be the producers of that space.*
>
> *Whether you own a home or a vacation spot or whatever, you make a room available on the Airbnb platform. Airbnb then matches that supply with consumers' needs and desires—people who have come to Airbnb looking to spend time in a property. That efficiency of not having to own and build the supply makes Airbnb a much more price-sensitive alternative for the consumer. What Airbnb is doing is what all platforms fundamentally do—acquire enough producers and enough consumers*

and then have their intelligence systems digitally match the needs of the consumer with the supply made by the producers.

In a previous chapter, I introduced you to Dr. Roy Schoenberg, a leading innovator in putting tech to work for providers and patients and the president and cofounder of Amwell. Roy has a deep understanding of platforms in that his company has deployed a digital care enablement platform called *Converge*. This platform integrates in-person, virtual, and automated care into the existing workflows that providers use daily. Roy uses terms such as "clinical brokerage engine" and "switchboard" to describe how the platform matches the best clinician to patients, with minimal wait times, and enables providers by referring them to automated and digital health programs. Like all true platforms, its open architecture allows for other vendor applications to participate. For our second example, consider Roy's explanation of the difference between Amazon the platform and the products it sells on its platform:

The platform under Amazon is that giant switchboard that allows manufacturers of goods to say "I have something to sell." It allows Amazon to catalog those goods and classify them in a way that people can discover them, then puts them in front of consumers, finds out if they want them, and if they do, Amazon facilitates the whole chain of electrons to get that piece of inventory from where it resides right now into the hands of consumers. That's the part that you don't see, right? You just see the product page and say, "Oh, it's there. I can buy it." There's a distinction to be made between the product you bought from Amazon and the entire platform that is Amazon, which brought that product to your attention. To me, viscerally, that's the best way I can explain a platform. In healthcare it gets more complicated because we know that the notion of acquisition of healthcare services is not really a consumer thing. It's more of a provider/prescription kind of thing, but still, the analogy remains.

The ultimate goal of platforms such as Amazon is to create a frictionless experience beginning with discovery, continuing through search, and ending with an actual transaction. This type of platform is what's known as an exchange platform, specifically a marketplace platform, and according to Vince and Randy, a marketplace platform has a three-step approach to its business model:

Step One: Curating Vendors
The platforms must identify reliable sellers who add value to their site in terms of selection, quality, price, etc.

Step Two: Attracting Customers
The more people a platform can attract, the more powerful it becomes. Customers provide a lot of content to a platform in terms of reviews, feedback, and recommendations, all of which are very helpful to other users as well as the vendors themselves. There is a snowball effect that happens as a platform acquires more customers. It's called the *network effect*—more consumers on a platform attract more vendors, which then attract more consumers, and so on. The platform becomes more valuable as each additional user joins it. This distinguishes its business model from more static or linear electronic sites.

Step Three: Matching Customer Needs to "Best Fit" Vendors
The more a customer uses a platform, the more a platform gets to "know" that customer. The platform can then suggest products and services that it knows the customer has already shown an interest in. Three implicit platform attributes include (1) ease of use, (2) transpar-

ency, and (3) options. The easier it is to navigate and use, the more transparent it is, and the more options it offers, the more likely a platform is to create the type of experience and "best fit" that attracts more consumers.

The core principle to remember here is that platforms are not just operating systems. The platform business model is different insofar as it competes and creates value in ways that traditional business models can't. As described in a *Deloitte Insights* report, "Traditional 'pipeline' businesses compete on cost, quality, and market breadth, and try to capture part of the value chain by focusing on economies of scale, unique intellectual property, specialized resources, geographic presence, and brand. They have traditionally used mergers and acquisitions (M&A) to grow and diversify. But alternatives such as platform-enabled ecosystems can help organizations improve and expand their services as they tap into the expertise of other organizations."[104]

CONNECTION AND COLLABORATION

When it comes to platforms, the whole is much greater than the sum of its parts. And the platform doesn't just represent a digital online analogue for a marketplace. It goes far beyond that to deliver an almost magical experience that's augmented by AI. It's kind of like all of the stores in the world, delivered online, on one site, providing you with a personalized, concierge-like shopping experience.

It's pretty clear that platforms facilitate a giant leap forward from how we interact in healthcare today, even taking into consideration the digital advances currently employed. For example, electronic

---

104 Simon Gisby et al., "New Business Model in Health Care: Building Platform-Enabled Ecosystems," *Deloitte Insights*, 2022, https://www2.deloitte.com/content/dam/insights/articles/us165009_chs-health-care-ecosystem/DI_CHS-Health-care-ecosystem.pdf.

health records are stored and shared digitally, but they are used in a very channeled and linear one-to-one manner. That's totally unlike a platform, which can host whole communities of vendors and consumers and provide consumer-grade transparency, options, and ease of use. For those of you who use your provider's or hospital's so-called "patient portal," how similar is that to Amazon's streaming entertainment experience? Not very. The patient portal doesn't allow you to compare providers or get detailed descriptions. You can't view what *others like you* chose. You can't compare prices or get options based on how much you're willing to spend. You can't even get your previous shopping history. And although patient portals are getting better, the customer experience is still pretty clunky. To be fair, patient portals and electronic medical records are a huge digital advance over paper charting, bringing critically important improvements in patient safety and quality, and billing. But they're still really dumb platforms. And it feels that way for providers as well as for patients. The next-gen healthcare platforms have robust infrastructure and network-building capabilities, in addition to an exceptional customer experience.

The one key attribute that distinguishes modern platforms is the "network effect." Think about how you as a patient might use a healthcare platform. You would be linked to your primary doctor through the platform. But you could also be connected to specialists, care management experts, healthcare navigators, health coaches, financial assistants, blood testing and medical imaging sites, and even your family members, as well as other patients who are going through similar experiences or with similar conditions. Let's say that all adds up to fourteen different stakeholders. The limits of our current digital, as well as nondigital, healthcare system force you to find each of these stakeholders' contact information and communicate with them one by one. If you did the math, your group of fourteen would have to communicate through ninety-one separate channels. That's a grossly inefficient, time-consuming, costly, and terribly frustrating transactional barrier.

By contrast, on a true platform, you would only have to initiate *one* communication to everyone because all fourteen people would already be linked on that platform. This is the network effect in action. Each new customer and each new vendor would make the platform more valuable by adding more resources, more options, more information—all of which enhances the network effect. If you're the one hundredth user, it's actually a lot better than being the first user, which is not true of traditional business models.

Finally, a platform enables you to customize your user experience as it gets to "know" your behaviors and preferences through multiple streams of data. Using sophisticated analytics, it predicts what you want and how you want it. That, in turn, keeps you coming back. In the case of healthcare, personalization can also be leveraged as a means of wayfinding—utilizing AI and analytics to help guide patients and healthcare consumers through potential next steps in their healthcare journey.

HOW THE PLATFORM BENEFITS STAKEHOLDERS

A "flywheel" is a platform strategy to build and sustain engagement by leveraging the customer experience. Many consider a flywheel to be a type of network effect. Perhaps the best-known Amazon flywheel is their Prime membership program, which, for an annual fee, provides fast and free shipping, access to their massive library of movies and TV shows, and other special deals and discounts. The mandate for the company is to make user interaction a "daily habit."

Keeping the flywheel metaphor in mind, Vince and Randy believe there are four factors that will drive long-term market adoption of healthcare platforms. Each factor represents a trend currently gathering strength in the market.

Value-Based Care and Payments

Platforms will lower the cost of care as they open the door for alternative payment models, as well as create competition within the current opaque FFS system. Vince has this to say about this particular flywheel factor: "We believe a health system on a platform model will be particularly ripe within value-based care approaches. If a patient could potentially be treated more efficiently or more effectively somewhere else, then the incentive may be to actually refer the patient to wherever that patient can receive the best care. Isn't that refreshing?"

Consumerism

As we discussed back in chapter 2, Americans want a similar experience in healthcare as they have with other facets of their consumer life. People want options and choices. They want unbiased information to be able to make comparisons. And they want trusted and expert guidance in navigating an often-serious set of decisions in a complex sector. In other words, they want to be informed and empowered. Healthcare consumers today are demanding this experience. Satisfying that demand is possible with a platform approach to healthcare.

Home-Based Care Ecosystem and Virtual Care

Platforms will greatly enhance home-based care and virtual care by providing all the current care options, updated regularly, but while you're at home or, frankly, anywhere you are connected to the internet.

Imagine a "streaming healthcare" system available to you 24/7, a platform that delivers a care experience with the best combined qualities of online shopping, online entertainment, and online communication. Platforms will greatly enable healthcare to shift beyond the concrete walls of clinics, urgent care centers, emergency departments, and hospitals.

Interoperability and Data Sharing

One of the great limitations of our current health system is lack of interoperability. Randy explains the current system this way: "It's a gatekeeper model where we have to seek care from the gatekeeper, instead of the gatekeeper steering us to services that are most relevant and valuable to us as consumers of that healthcare. Our data is captured in a silo and is very hard for us to access, let alone for other providers who we're interacting with." One of the most powerful capabilities of a platform is its capacity to connect stakeholders and share information selectively. The platform shifts the notion of an electronic medical record beyond its current digital walls—transitioning control into the hands of the consumer so that accessing, sharing, communicating, and consulting are free and easily available options.

IMPLICATIONS FOR HEALTHCARE LEADERS

Judging from our experience in other industries, platforms are likely to be the next game changer in healthcare—a 'beyond the walls' catalyst. All of the trends, movements, and market forces we discuss in this book can be integrated into, connected by, and greatly enabled by platforms. Platforms will connect all of our digital interactions, greatly advance virtual care, and elevate home-based care. Elderly and frail seniors can be connected much more seamlessly to their health systems, to caregivers, and to friends and family. And contextual, whole-person health can be integrated much more easily through platforms.

If you're a healthcare leader, you might wonder how all of this will impact your planning. This is how Vince believes you should think about it:

> *I'll quickly summarize a good, better, and best framework for thinking about platforms if you're an incumbent. "Good" is that you don't have to throw out your existing business model. You can experiment and start thinking about building a platform strategy around some of your existing technology platforms, such as your patient portal. "Better" requires a little bit of a leap in conceptualization, but you can begin thinking about the business as being a platform. And the third level, "Best" is taking an ecosystem approach where you get to the point of including your competitors, but you don't have to own every piece of the system. You can build an asset-light business model. I think we'll see a lot more specialization in healthcare as companies recognize that they don't have to do it all themselves.*

What's the risk of not entering this bold new era? The fact that many others are waiting to dive in. Sara Vaezy is executive VP and chief strategy and digital officer at Providence, where she is responsible for digital strategy, product innovation, marketing, digital experience, and commercialization for the integrated delivery network, which includes fifty-two hospitals and over one thousand clinics serving over five

Judging from our experience in other industries, platforms are likely to be the next game changer in healthcare.

million patients. Healthcare platforms are a priority for her because she believes if healthcare companies aren't proactive in embracing this technology, the results could be problematic. In our podcast conversation, she bluntly described what could happen to those that hesitate to make this move:

> *They're going to chip away at our profitable businesses. It may not be that Amazon or Walmart or CVS or Walgreens or whoever will deliver a single death blow, but they're going to collectively chip away at the already deteriorating kind of margins of health systems and take away what little profitable business that we have. Health systems can't survive and remain viable that way. The second thing that's going to happen is that we're going to become downstream price takers, pushed into only those businesses like hospital services that we can provide—services these entities aren't going to want to take on because they are very operationally challenging and very expensive to run. We will become commoditized services that only compete on the basis of price. And that's a bad place to be.*

This is one of the reasons that the introduction of platforms into healthcare is a *burning* issue. New platform entities are offering a superior patient experience and value proposition, controlling the basic business models, and diverting revenue streams and margins. While platforms have not yet become mainstream in healthcare delivery, we do have some examples that are making inroads.

EARLY ADOPTERS

Now that we've explored the idea of platforms and their potential for transforming healthcare delivery, let's go from theory to reality and examine two innovative companies who are bringing this idea to life, Transcarent and Uber Health.

Transcarent: Creating a "One-Stop Shop"

In chapter 2 I introduced you to Glen Tullman, one of the most successful healthcare entrepreneurs and investors of our era. Over the past couple of decades, he's been at the helm of a string of industry-leading healthcare tech companies and over the past nine years has coled a remarkable VC firm, 7wireVentures, with his partner, Lee Shapiro. Glen has always been a huge proponent of transforming healthcare through technology. In fact, one of his favorite quotes comes from science fiction writer Arthur C. Clarke's third law: "Any sufficiently advanced technology is indistinguishable from magic." But there's another law that comes into play here, and that's the law of unintended consequences. Ironically, digital technology has created a new set of problems in the healthcare industry in that there are now a multitude of fragmented digital healthcare solutions. So many, in fact, that it's become near impossible for providers to assess, curate, and integrate them. For example, there are hundreds of digital solutions for chronic conditions such as diabetes or depression, and these solutions are stand-alones that don't communicate or coordinate with one another. Glen captures the frustration like this: "We keep seeing that, instead of trying to solve their customers' problems, healthcare people just keep throwing technology at it."

The truth is that this situation is overwhelming for patients as well as providers, with the impact being contrary to the intention of improving and simplifying the consumer experience of care delivery. This is why Glen has turned to a platform approach as the ideal solution for connecting the myriad devices, apps, and services within a consumer-friendly ecosystem. With his latest venture, Transcarent, Glen's goal is to create a viable alternative for large self-insured employers who are seeking a high-value, cost-effective, easily accessible, and easy-to-navigate healthcare system for their employees. Transcarent resembles a concierge medical practice. The "magic" Glen is attempting to pull off is to organize everything around employees' healthcare needs using virtual, automated, and in-person care.

So what does it look like? Let's say your employer signs you up for Transcarent's services. The first thing you do is download their app, which opens up a portal to an interconnected menu of care options. You can connect with care navigators, health coaches, pharmacists, physical therapists, your primary care doctor, specialists, and so on. One consumer promise is that you can be connected to a provider within sixty seconds. Whatever your problem is, they'll help you identify the next best step rather than you having to navigate the complexities of the healthcare system on your own. Glen said, "We want three things from healthcare. First, we want unbiased information … and options. Then the next thing we want is trusted guidance. Then finally, we want access. What we want to do in Transcarent is bring the same transparency [and access] to everybody."

Why is Glen targeting his platform at employers? Because he believes self-insured employers are going to be major drivers of the changes that need to happen in the healthcare system, as he puts it, "If you look at the key players, there are large payers, there are large PBMs, and there are large health systems. But no one is actually advocating for the stakeholders who are actually paying the bills, and those are self-insured employers and all of us."

Of all the stakeholders in healthcare, Glen believes it's the employers and individual consumers who are most incentivized to bring down costs, improve outcomes, and improve the consumer care experience. Even the federal government is conflicted because politicians in Congress are courted and their campaigns funded by incredibly powerful, well-funded lobbying groups, such as the pharmaceutical industry's Pharma, and the health insurance industry's trade association, AHIP.

A few years ago, I interviewed Aaron Martin, an executive at Amazon who had crossed over into healthcare to join Providence Health and is now back at Amazon, leading its healthcare division. He shared the Amazon platform playbook, which is pretty straightforward. There are two important stakeholders in any industry: the consumer and the provider. What Amazon has done in other industries, such as publishing, is to cut out the many middlemen. That's pretty much how I would sum up Glen's consumerist platform playbook. Transcarent's value proposition is to reduce the complexity and escalating costs of the current system by eliminating the numerous middlemen and connecting patients directly to providers on a seamless, coordinated, and transparent platform of care.

While Transcarent is still in its early days, there are some encouraging results in terms of reductions in unnecessary emergency visits, reductions in readmissions, and a reduction in total costs of care.

One core element of Transcarent is curation, which is a critical success factor for any platform. They have a real shot at providing a variety of high-quality, lower-cost options by curating those that demonstrate the best and most reliable outcomes and consumer experiences. Glen sums up the Transcarent platform vision this way: "Amazon is an 'experience' company. Apple is an 'experience' company. We're an 'experience' company. We'll use technology, we'll use data science, we'll use everything we can to create this amazing experience where you say, 'You know what, there wasn't a time when I didn't feel informed and in control.' And that's what we want for our healthcare experience."

Uber Health: A Transportation Platform

In describing Transcarent, Glen made numerous comparisons to how Uber transformed the transportation sector. Uber—a shining example of a successful platform business model—is now seeking to positively disrupt healthcare through their Uber Health division that launched about five years ago. The inflection point came when they hired Caitlin Donovan as the Global Head of Uber Health in 2021. In speaking with Caitlin, it's immediately apparent that she is brilliant and bold. She holds a degree in economics from Harvard and brings a deep hands-on experience, having held chief operating roles at numerous health tech and healthcare transportation companies. I had the privilege of interviewing both her and Dr. Mike Cantor, the Uber Health Chief Medical Officer, who is both a practicing geriatrician and attorney and has held leadership roles at Bright Health Plan, Care-Centrix, and the New England Quality Care Alliance (NEQCA)—the physician network for Tufts Medical Center in Boston.

Now, you may wonder what part Uber can play in our healthcare system. It turns out to be a critically important one. The national average "no-show" rate for medical appointments is roughly 18 percent, which translates to almost one in five visits.[105] According to Caitlin, those missed appointments cost the healthcare industry about $150 billion a year. Remember, we're not just talking about appointments with primary care physicians and specialists. We're talking about appointments for radiation therapy, chemotherapy, hemodialysis, intravenous infusion therapies, CT scans, MRIs, and so on. Once a patient misses one of these appointments, that slot is gone forever, and so is the revenue that would have been created. And importantly,

---

105 Parviz Kheirkhah et al. "Prevalence, Predictors and Economic Consequences of No-Shows," *BMC Health Services Research* 16, no. 13 (January 14, 2016). https://doi:10.1186/s12913-015-1243-z.

patients don't receive the healthcare they were scheduled to receive, which translates into a negative impact on health outcomes at both the individual and population levels. It's a massive problem from the care access perspective, the financial perspective, and the clinical outcomes perspective.

Uber Health is out to fix this multifaceted problem by tapping into the

> The national average "no-show" rate for medical appointments is roughly 18 percent, which translates to almost one in five visits.

logistics of Uber. Since its launch, they've worked to improve access to non-emergency medical transportation (NEMT) and have continued expanding its platform to meet the needs of plans, providers, and patients—including grocery, meals, home testing, and medication delivery. In addition to patient-focused transportation, they're also working with healthcare workers and providers to transport them to their place of service. Through this assortment of healthcare-related services, they are able to address social determinants of health factors as well as contextual care issues that may be preventing patients from achieving successful treatments and recovery. Recall in chapter 5 the story of the woman who couldn't get to her dialysis treatments because she also had to transport a child she was caring for to their doctor appointments. Uber Health firmly believes it can solve that type of situation more efficiently and effectively than the patchwork network of vendors most healthcare systems are currently deploying. How? Through the use of one of the most sophisticated, tech-enabled transportation platforms in the world: Uber.

Caitlin offers a compelling example of how healthcare systems can literally save thousands of dollars and, more importantly, lives, simply by working with Uber Health to transport patients.

"Just to give one really concrete example of what happens if you don't fix the structure of the system, there's a really interesting, true anecdote that happened a couple of months ago, where we had a relationship with a payer and one of their risk-bearing providers. They had a patient, who is a dual eligible member [eligible for both Medicare and Medicaid] and had to cross state lines to get a medical service that they needed frequently. Medicaid wouldn't pay for the transportation, because the care was being delivered in a different state. And, because it happened so frequently, the patient had already exhausted their Medicare benefit. With Uber, the round trip would cost about $80 to see their physician. However, the insurance company wouldn't do it because the benefit didn't technically exist. The patient ended up having an acute event and called an ambulance. The cost of transportation alone was thousands of dollars versus the $80 we quoted and the patient ended up in the hospital."

Michael asks the poignant question:

"Why not spend the $80 upfront, get this person to the service they need, avoid an acute worsening of their condition and exacerbation, which then leads to a very costly and risky hospitalization?"

Uber Health is also far more than just a transport service for patients. They intend to act as a "wraparound" for someone's health-care journey. What does that mean? It means their services can improve the whole experience. They're able to transport healthcare workers such as nurses and home aides who won't have to use their own car or public transportation, nor worry about finding parking if that happens to be an issue. The patient can thereby be assured of help arriving in a timely and reliable fashion.

When Uber Health is working directly with a provider or healthcare system, it also cuts through enormous amounts of red tape regarding benefits management. The steps required to obtain transportation services for any given patient can slow down and even prevent those services from being obtained. Say you're a medical assistant, nurse, or medical office worker and you need to schedule transportation for a patient. You'll have to look up that person's insurance, call the benefits manager, and talk to them about what the specific insurance plan covers and doesn't cover. Then you have to call a specific medical-use-only transportation company to set it up. That's a huge amount of time and energy spent to simply set up a ride. In addition to that, many of these programs also require a three-day advance notice, which makes them less flexible for patients and providers who may need to get someone home or to a clinic sooner.

In contrast, Uber Health has created a platform with the healthcare ecosystem in mind that automatically retrieves patients' insurance benefits information. The HIPAA-compliant platform interacts with the medical office and healthcare system's software so any patient's specific insurance benefit can be accessed at the point transportation is being scheduled. Uber Health's platform continues to make it simple for both medical staff and patients (regardless of access to a smartphone) by allowing care coordinators to schedule the appointment pickup and drop-off while notifying patients of updates to their ride through either text messaging or a phone call.

For many patients, convenient and affordable access to transportation is, in fact, a matter of life and death. Michael talks about an innovative program Uber is piloting that demonstrates how transportation can directly address one of the most serious healthcare disparities in America.

"... we did a trial, a small study in Washington, D.C. with pregnant people who lived in geographically remote parts of D.C.—where they had to travel an hour by public transportation to get to their prenatal maternal health visits. We were able to identify through our partnership with Surgo Ventures where those people lived, who they were, and who was at the highest risk of maternal poor outcomes. We were able to then offer them rides. One interesting question was—should their provider order the transportation or should we just give transport vouchers to the pregnant people, and let them schedule themselves? We discovered that offering both options helped meet the varying needs and preferences of pregnant people. In fact, 75 percent of them said that it would have taken them more time to get to their appointments without this program. On average, participants reported they saved one hour per appointment with this program compared to other transportation options. That makes a big difference in the health of those pregnant folks and their babies, in terms of also ensuring that they get to well-baby visits and their own check-ups after delivery as well. The technology makes it scalable, accessible, and affordable."

The program for pregnant women Michael is talking about is called "Rides for Moms," and it's a boon for low-income high-risk patients in the Washington, DC, area. A lot of these patients might not have shown up for their appointments because of the time involved and the difficulty inherent in the old system. Think about the human and financial costs when a high-risk pregnancy ends up in a bad outcome or with a baby in a neonatal ICU. The monetary costs for a single neonatal ICU stay can be tens of thousands of dollars. Imagine if the Rides for Moms program was implemented on a national scale. It would have the potential to improve lives, save lives, dramatically reduce avoidable costs of care, and address one of the most heartbreaking healthcare disparities in the US.

Just as Amazon started as an online bookstore, Uber began as a simple ride-for-hire service. Now, its Health arm has evolved into a platform that can serve patients directly where they live, by either taking them to where they receive care or delivering food, medicine, and even healthcare workers to their homes.

Final Thoughts

Uber, Transcarent, and others are real-life examples of platforms that are shifting healthcare beyond the walls of its legacy constraints. They're making healthcare far more convenient, accessible, and affordable by providing choices and by creating connections. Over the past decade, so many facets of our lives have literally been transformed by the power of platforms, and we are beginning to witness the same occur within healthcare.

Here's a final message from Dr. Randy Williams, whom we met at the beginning of this chapter:

> *If we don't get anything else across in our discussions with healthcare provider executives, we at least want them to recognize that platform thinking is something you need to embrace and get familiar with because other very large, very well-capitalized entities are coming for your patients. Second, as you think about platforms, recognize that having a digital infrastructure enables you, but it isn't a destination. The destination is thinking about how value can be unlocked and provided to your healthcare consumers, as in a platform. One last point: we're not encouraging every healthcare organization to become a platform business model, but we certainly*

want you to be informed enough about it to actually weigh the question strategically and come to a conclusion about it.

In the next chapter, we're going to explore the "Titans of Disruption." These are mammoth brands that are out to radically improve healthcare delivery at scale.

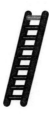

CHAPTER 8

THE TITANS OF DISRUPTION

When large successful companies see an opportunity, they move into it, and they don't move small. They move big.

—Dr. Robert Pearl, professor, Stanford University, Schools of Medicine and Business

Regarding *Titans*, the actual reference here is to the powerful deities in Greek mythology known as the Titans, who preceded the Olympian gods. Cronus, Prometheus, and Atlas are some of the Titans' names you may recall. The actions of these Titans had an outsize effect on what happened on earth and on the natural order of the world. In the same vein, the actions of the large stakeholders we're going to explore in this chapter are having an outsize impact on our healthcare world, and they are setting the stage for the next generation of industry-leading stakeholders in healthcare.

SECTION 1: THE GAME PLAN

Huge retail giants such as Amazon and Walmart as well as massive pharmacy chains such as Walgreens and CVS are well-known entities. These titans of disruption have transformed and dominated the retail and pharmacy industries. Over the past few years, they've been bringing their innovative consumer-oriented capabilities into the domain of healthcare delivery. What may seem like episodic market splashes to most people is actually a highly strategic, well-resourced, consistent, multiyear march to transform healthcare delivery. This should come as no surprise to anyone. The healthcare industry now makes up nearly one-fifth of the US economy. And while there have been faltering steps along the way, what these titans are particularly adept at is learning and pivoting and bringing resources to bear that are orders of magnitude greater than what the majority of legacy stakeholders in the healthcare industry are capable of. And to be clear, what we're talking about here is not a recent development. I first wrote about these titans in *Reframing Healthcare*, published in 2019. Based on over a decade of industry tracking, I offer five high-level observations that may not be apparent to the casual observer.

1. The Titans of Disruption are highly attuned to consumers' needs.

Their healthcare rhetoric and approach has been incredibly consumer oriented. These are the most skilled and scaled retailers. They've been listening to what consumers (and the market) have been saying about the deficiencies in American healthcare delivery—really listening. One example of this comes from Karen Lynch, previously an Aetna executive, who led a massive healthcare consumer-input gathering initiative a few years back. She subsequently became CEO of CVS Health, the result of a merger of CVS and Aetna. When I first read the Aetna consumer health report Lynch led, I was beyond impressed. I had never heard of a company declaring so boldly and so explicitly the importance of discovering what people actually wanted from healthcare. Yes, hospitals and provider groups were asking patients for feedback on their experience of hospitals and clinics, but that's a world of difference from asking people what they actually *need and want* from healthcare. We, in legacy healthcare, had been asking people what they *thought about us*. Karen and her colleagues were asking people what they *wanted from us*. I not only appreciate the difference but also recognize its disruptive potential. All of these titans of disruption are bringing their decades of consumer expertise to bear in order to learn what their customers want from their healthcare, what problems they need solved, and how they want care to be delivered. This makes sense, as it's the only way these new entrants can provide an effective and desirable alternative.

2. Their pace of disruption is accelerating.

When I first began tracking these companies, earthshaking announcements were occurring at a frequency of, perhaps, once every two to three years. Fast-forward and the tempo is now measured in weeks to months. For example, CVS has made eighteen major healthcare acquisitions, with seven occurring in the last five years.[106] The newly merged entity, CVS Health—formed in 2018—steadily continued to expand its role into care delivery with the launch of its HealthHUBs in 2019, SuperClinics in 2021, and the acquisitions of home health provider Signify Health in 2022, which was finalized in 2023 along with a second acquisition in 2023 of Medicare Advantage primary care provider Oak Street Health. Amazon had not made any major

---

106 Claire Wallace, "9 Fast Facts on CVS Health Acquisitions," Becker's ASC Review, September 6, 2022, https://www.beckersasc.com/asc-news/9-fast-facts-on-cvs-health-acquisitions.html.

plays into healthcare until it launched Haven in 2018. But since then it has launched its own care delivery through Amazon Care in 2020, rebranded its online pharmacy as Amazon Pharmacy in 2020, and acquired the national primary care physician practice, One Medical, in 2023.[107, 108] One large national tech retailer that has been flying under the radar, but just came out as a new entrant in healthcare delivery, is Best Buy. Best Buy has made a number of significant acquisitions in the healthcare space, in rapid succession since 2018, when it first acquired personal emergency response company GreatCall.[109]

3. They are getting bolder.

I'm not sure when I first noticed the shift, but both the tone and the narrative has significantly transformed over the past decade. It used to be that their narrative conveyed a scoped intention to fill the gaps in care delivery—to work in-between and around providers and hospital systems. This prior rhetoric skirted the notion of direct competition. Then came a sort of tipping point. It was a marked revision from "we're not going to take any of your business away" to "we're going to do this better and therefore earn the right to care for patients by providing more convenient care at lower cost with better quality." If you carefully follow their progression, the increasingly apparent intention describes a plan to create national healthcare platforms and to provide care across the spectrum.

---

107   Leila Hawkins, "Amazon's Move to Healthcare—a Timeline," Healthcare Digital, July 7, 2021, https://healthcare-digital.com/technology-and-ai/amazons-move-healthcare-timeline.

108   Lydia Ramsey Pflanzer, "Amazon Has Been Trying to Break into Healthcare for Years. Here's a Look at Everything It's Done," Insider, February 15, 2023, https://www.businessinsider.com/amazon-healthcare-rxpass-pharmacy-clinic-one-medical.

109   "Best Buy Acquires GreatCall, a Leading Connected Health Services Provider," Best Buy, August 15, 2018, https://investors.bestbuy.com/investor-relations/news-and-events/financial-releases/news-details/2018/Best-Buy-Acquires-GreatCall-a-Leading-Connected-Health-Services-Provider/default.aspx.

Karen Lynch from CVS Health has been explicit about just this aim in remarks she made at the 2022 JPMorgan conference: "We will further build out our primary care offerings to guide consumers across the entire care continuum…. It also will represent a shift for us to risk-based primary care versus the traditional models of fee for service primary care."[110]

Roz Brewer, CEO of Walgreens, has also described that company's strategy to consolidate all of Walgreens healthcare delivery assets into a single platform, Walgreens Health, as a precursor to caring for healthcare needs across the continuum. In an interview in 2022, Brewer said, "This platform will create an integrated experience for consumers across their journey and knit together the products and services from Walgreens Health and our partners."[111]

Walmart got into retail care delivery early, in the mid-2000s, with in-store clinics run by hospitals. But it was a decade later when their rhetoric noticeably shifted, and they began demonstrating a commitment to becoming predominant providers of care. In 2014 Walmart launched its first company-owned care clinic and then in 2018 its first Healthcare Services Super Center,[112, 113] causing some industry

110   Matthew Weinstock, "Three Healthcare Trends to Watch," Oliver Wyman, 2022, https://www.oliverwyman.com/our-expertise/perspectives/health/2022/jan/three-healthcare-trends-to-watch-.html.

111   Tom Sullivan, "Walgreens CEO Roz Brewer on Improving the Patient Care Journey," Health Evolution, February 9, 2022, https://www.healthevolution.com/insider/walgreens-ceo-roz-brewer-on-improving-the-patient-care-journey/.

112   Katrina Rossos, "Walmart Care Clinics: Thinking outside the Big Box," *Pharmacy Times* 80, no. 10 (October 2014), https://www.pharmacytimes.com/view/walmart-care-clinics-thinking-outside-the-big-box.

113   Bruce Japsen, "Walmart's First Healthcare Services 'Super Center' Opens," *Forbes*, September 13, 2019, https://www.forbes.com/sites/brucejapsen/2019/09/13/walmarts-first-healthcare-services-super-center-opens/.

experts to predict that Walmart could become the biggest PCP in the country.[114]

4. They are vertically integrating and rapidly acquiring capabilities and customers.

Unlike hospital systems that have been merging horizontally—that is, merging with other hospital systems to spread geographically—these titans of disruption are merging vertically. They've been acquiring complementary assets and capabilities and testing them in the market for years now. They are focusing on a broad swath of the continuum of care, including primary care, postacute care, chronic disease management, home-based care, virtual care, behavioral health, care management, care navigation, pharmacy, specialty pharmacy services, and durable medical equipment. To date, with rare exception, they are not providing brick-and-mortar, hospital-based care. Their vertical integration approach may be a function of being relatively new entrants to healthcare and needing to rapidly amass a broad set of capabilities. But I suspect there's more to it than that.

Vertical integration brings with it a much more rapid pace of change than attempting to build capabilities on one's own, which is the typical approach legacy healthcare systems have taken. Buying (versus building) also brings viable businesses on board with new customers, additional growth channels, and importantly, immediate revenue streams. One example of the colossal impact of vertical integration was when CVS acquired Aetna in 2018, in a $69 billion deal that was (and still is) the largest healthcare acquisition in market history. The announcement sent unprecedented shock waves through-

---

114   Sai Balasubramanian, "Walmart Continues Its Rapid Expansion in Healthcare, Announcing 16 New Facilities," *Forbes,* October 27, 2022, https://www.forbes.com/sites/saibala/2022/10/27/walmart-continues-its-rapid-expansion-in-healthcare-announcing-16-new-facilities/.

out the industry. Reports from that time called it a "transformative moment" that "marked the start of a new day in healthcare."[115]

5. They are much larger with less fixed costs.

When we compare these companies with legacy healthcare systems, we can see one obvious strategic advantage and one that may be less obvious. What's obvious is that these companies have significantly more financial resources. What's not as obvious is that they have far less fixed infrastructure costs (a.k.a. hospitals).

Take a look at the graph below comparing the revenues and revenue growth of businesses between 2019 and 2022. As you can see, only the UnitedHealthcare Group is really in the same neighborhood as Amazon, Walmart, and CVS Health and that Group earns most of its revenue from its health insurance arm. The hospital-based healthcare systems pale in comparison, and these represent some of the largest hospital-based care delivery systems in the country.

115 Eli Richman, "CVS Closes $69B Acquisition of Aetna in a 'Transformative Moment' for the Industry," *Fierce Healthcare*, November 28, 2018, https://www.fiercehealthcare.com/payer/cvs-closes-69-billion-acquisition-aetna; "CVS Health Completes Acquisition of Aetna, Marking Start of Transforming Consumer Health Experience," Cision PR Newswire, November 28, 2018, https://www.prnewswire.com/news-releases/cvs-health-completes-acquisition-of-aetna-marking-start-of-transforming-consumer-health-experience-300756921.html.

PANDEMIC HELPED DRIVE DOUBLE DIGIT GROWTH FOR HEALTHCARE GIANTS, EXCEPT FOR HEALTH SYSTEMS

Revenues of Largest Health Systems Grew at Only Five Percent Annually

Annual Revenue of Largest Healthcare Companies and Health Systems
BILLIONS OF DOLLARS

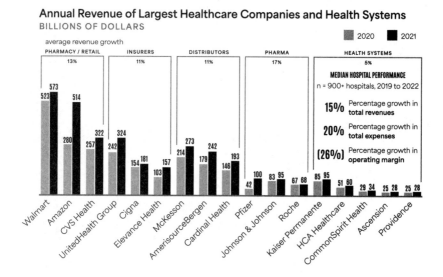

Source: A battle of (growing) titans in healthcare; Gist Healthcare, Feb. 24, 2023, https://gisthealthcare.com/a-battle-of-growing-titans-in-healthcare/

These companies generate revenues that are orders of magnitude greater than hospital-based systems which among other things, allows them to invest in further growth.. And despite their size, they're highly adaptive and agile from a consumer perspective, a logistics perspective, and a technical perspective. As a result of their vertical acquisitions, they have a diversified portfolio of revenue streams and payment models, which creates a resilience factor you don't see in hospital-based healthcare systems.

THE SHORT, MIDDLE, AND LONG GAME

Dr. Robert Pearl was the CEO of the Permanente Medical Group from 1999 to 2017 and has been named one of Modern Healthcare's 50 most influential physician leaders. He currently serves as a clinical professor of surgery at Stanford University School of Medicine and is on the faculty of the Stanford Graduate School of Business. He has authored two books, *Mistreated: Why We Think We're Getting Good Health Care—and Why We're Usually Wrong* and *Uncaring: How the Culture of Medicine Kills Doctors and Patients*. Dr. Pearl also hosts a podcast called *Fixing Healthcare* and is a regular contributor to *Forbes*. He is one of the most accomplished, thoughtful, and analytic leaders I've had the opportunity to speak with. Robbie recently authored an online *Forbes* piece that resonates with my own thinking in explaining the highly strategic actions of these titans of disruption.[116] As a guest on my podcast, he elaborated on the long-term disruptive strategies of these organizations.

> *What I see is a short game, a middle game, and a long game. The short game is what they're playing right now. Acquire the pieces to be able to dominate each of these three areas [pharmacy, insurance, clinics and physicians]. The middle game, and we're seeing it already, is moving into the one part of American healthcare that is fully capitated. That is Medicare Advantage. Each of these companies has millions of Medicare Advantage patients now and sees that as a major growth area.*
>
> *Once you can show your ability to take a set payment, which is what a capitation is for a population of people, and reduce the*

---

116   Robert Pearl, "Amazon, CVS, Walmart Are Playing Healthcare's Long Game," *Forbes*, October 10, 2022, https://www.forbes.com/sites/robertpearl/2022/10/10/amazon-cvs-walmart-are-playing-healthcares-long-game/.

inefficiencies as well as take out the wasted expense, you have a very strong value proposition that you can now take to the payers of care, the businesses and individuals, and potentially even the government. I see a ten-year horizon in which these large retailers will move into healthcare the same way they moved into a broad swath of the retail world. I could see them displacing and eliminating many of the current independent insurers, many of the physicians and hospitals, and many of the smaller pharmaceutical drugstore chains.

The long game, from Robbie's perspective, is market domination. Once these titans have pharmacies, clinics, and providers as well as the insurance arm *and* can leverage their size and customer reach to attract self-funded businesses, they can create economies of scale that lead to a self-perpetuating upward trajectory of value and growth. This "supersystem" starts with lower costs and more convenient healthcare that attracts more customers, thereby creating more revenue and profit and a greater capacity to build and scale.

These titans will leverage three major capabilities. First, they have a highly developed consumer orientation with a focus on convenient access, customer service, reliability, and low cost. Second, they are building their own care ecosystems, bit by bit, carving out significant chunks of consumers' healthcare needs. Third, as Robbie points out, their goal is to take value-based or risk-based payments to become masters of capitation. Risk-based payment aligns with their business models, given that many of them either have or are acquiring insurance capabilities. That's a significant advantage over the majority of hospital-based healthcare systems.

SECTION 2: THE RETAILERS

Part of the disruptive potential of these titans is that they're so diversified they defy categorization. They don't fit neatly into the provider bucket or the payer bucket. And they have additional business lines such as retail, pharmacy, pharmacy benefit management, healthcare management services, data analytics, and cloud computing services. So what do we call them? Left with what is an imperfect categorization, let's start with what I will label the "retailer" category.

> Part of the disruptive potential of these titans is that they're so diversified they defy categorization.

Amazon

The following graphic offers a quick overview of what Amazon has done to date in the healthcare field.[117]

Amazon's massive size, its commitment to resourcing and developing healthcare services, combined with its expertise at serving consumers, make it one of the most powerful disruptors. Here are some of the biggest moves Amazon has made to build its healthcare brand and platform in recent years. In 2018 Amazon acquired prescription delivery company PillPack and then in 2020 relaunched PillPack as part of Amazon Pharmacy. In that year they also launched their own primary care services through Amazon Care. In 2022 they partnered with an online behavioral company, Ginger.io, to offer remote behavioral health services through Amazon Care. And in 2023

---

117   Lisa Bielamowicz, "Toward a Platform Future," presentation, October 12, 2023, Group Practice Improvement Network (GPIN) Symposium.

they finalized the deal for the purchase of One Medical and shuttered Amazon Care.

AMAZON ASSEMBLING CONTINUUM OF HEALTH SOLUTION

Amazon's proposed acquisition of One Medical provides a brick-and-mortar footprint along with thousands of employer relationships, something it struggled to achieve through Amazon Care

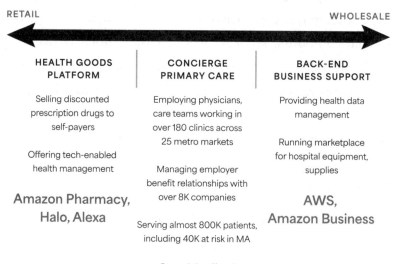

One Medical Acquisition Provides Amazon a Missing Customer Base

RETAIL ← → WHOLESALE

HEALTH GOODS PLATFORM	CONCIERGE PRIMARY CARE	BACK-END BUSINESS SUPPORT
Selling discounted prescription drugs to self-payers	Employing physicians, care teams working in over 180 clinics across 25 metro markets	Providing health data management
Offering tech-enabled health management	Managing employer benefit relationships with over 8K companies	Running marketplace for hospital equipment, supplies
Amazon Pharmacy, Halo, Alexa	Serving almost 800K patients, including 40K at risk in MA	**AWS, Amazon Business**
	One Medical	

The One Medical acquisition is fascinating. For starters, it's a great example of the buy versus build approach. Amazon had initially begun to develop its own hybrid primary care service, but once it acquired One Medical, Amazon shuttered the build option and placed its bet on the buy-and-rapidly-scale approach. One Medical is a hybrid primary care model that includes (1) brick-and-mortar consumer/retail-oriented clinics; (2) virtual care, both synchronous and asynchronous; and (3) a highly networked healthcare navigation and consumer service. Basically, it's an entire primary care ecosystem that is available through an app but with the elegance and presence of a local concierge primary care chain.

In addition, One Medical acquired Iora Health a couple of years ago. Iora is one of the prototypical clinical leaders in Medicare Advantage–based (value-based) payment and a company that trailblazed contextualized, personalized care delivery. So with this one acquisition, Amazon has a national platform for one of the most technologically sophisticated and consumer-oriented Primary Care groups in the country, plus one of the most respected senior care, value-based provider groups.

That's the magic of vertical integration. In addition to building out its care pathway, Amazon has garnered significant attention for its cloud service, AWS. AWS offers cloud-based services as well as other business support to healthcare systems across the country, creating relationships and building another diversified set of healthcare capabilities. A 2022 report from KLAS research foundation said that health systems are choosing AWS over others such as Google or Microsoft because "they believe it's the most mature and healthcare-focused cloud platform" and "it was the fastest and most comprehensive cloud platform at the time."[118]

Amazon is not *just* about customer service. It's *all* about customer service. Its mission statement is "to be Earth's most customer-centric company."[119] They don't just have a consumer experience division; thanks to Jeff Bezos's vision, their entire organization is a consumer experience division whose goal is "to focus on delighting customers."[120] Amazon has fourteen leadership principles they adhere

118   Katie Adams, "Report: What Is Helping AWS Beat Its Health Cloud Competitors," *MedCity News*, June 7, 2022, https://medcitynews.com/2022/06/report-what-is-helping-aws-beat-its-health-cloud-competitors/.

119   "About Amazon," Amazon.com, accessed May 3, 2023, https://amazon.jobs/en/landing_pages/about-amazon.

120   Ibid.

to with religious fervor, the number one principle being "consumer obsession."[121] Consumer obsession has sadly not been a hallmark of our legacy healthcare system.

There's one more attribute that's critical to Amazon's success. As we discussed in chapter 7, platforms are already revolutionizing healthcare delivery, and Amazon is one of the earliest and most significant market platforms in existence. Amazon doesn't produce most of what they sell, but it has an incredibly sophisticated platform for marketing and selling. And in the same way that they revolutionized retail, they can use their market-leading platform to sell all sorts of healthcare services and products to consumers anywhere, anytime. I strongly suspect we're going to see the Amazon healthcare platform become a significant part of that company's online retail presence as well as a daily part of our lives.

Walmart

Similar to Amazon, Walmart is making major inroads into healthcare through both partnering and building. Transcarent, a platform we discussed in the last chapter, has partnered with Walmart to bring healthcare to self-funded employers. Walmart uses the documentation and billing services provided by the leading electronic medical records company Epic, which connects patient records across all of its healthcare services, including virtual care and pharmacy. And speaking of virtual care, in 2021 Walmart acquired MeMD, a telehealth service. In 2022 Walmart announced a ten-year partnership with UnitedHealthcare Optum, offering Optum's Medicare Advantage value-based insurance plans as well as its care management services to Walmart

---

customers.[122] Finally, Walmart has been rapidly expanding various forms of health clinics since it opened its first self-owned clinic in 2014. Currently, the company has thirty-two standalone Walmart health centers with plans to expand to seventy-seven by 2024.[123] This is in addition to their other in-store clinics and health "super centers."

The Walmart health story runs a lot deeper and begins much earlier than its recent acquisitions, partnerships, and clinics. Walmart began studying the healthcare costs of its employees well over a decade ago. The first thing they discovered was that healthcare was costing them a lot. The second thing they discovered was significant variation in costs for the same services. And the third thing they discovered was a tremendous and unexplained variation in the frequency with which different providers performed high-cost, relatively common procedures, such as hip and knee replacements, back surgeries, heart procedures, and cancer treatments. Here are some rough numbers I gleaned through conversations with Walmart execs over the years. At the time this data was provided to me, Walmart had over one million employees and dependents. Their annual healthcare costs were $4 billion. They discovered that by reducing inappropriate or unnecessary surgical procedures, they were able to save $1 billion a year (nearly 25 percent) in direct medical expenditures and somewhere between $2 billion and $3 billion overall from lost productivity and employee turnover. When they directed their employees to so-called medical "Centers of Excellence," they saw a 25 to 50 percent reduction in inappropriate surgeries, a 90 percent reduction in inappropriate back

---

122 "Walmart and UnitedHealth Group Collaborate to Deliver Access to High-Quality, Affordable Health Care," Walmart, September 7, 2022, https://corporate.walmart.com/newsroom/2022/09/07/walmart-and-unitedhealth-group-collaborate-to-deliver-access-to-high-quality-affordable-health-care.

123 David Carmouce, "Walmart Health Nearly Doubles in Size with Launch into Two New States in 2024," Walmart, March 2, 2023, https://corporate.walmart.com/newsroom/2023/03/02/walmart-health-nearly-doubles-in-size-with-launch-into-two-new-states-in-2024.

surgeries, and approximately 50 percent of their employees' cancer treatments were revised.[124]

This last point is critical to understanding the importance of Centers of Excellence to employers. It's not just about excellence in quality, outcomes, and experience. The single biggest distinguishing factor about Centers of Excellence is not the surgeries they do but the surgeries they *don't* do. They are highly selective about only operating when it's necessary. In addition to adopting a Centers of Excellence approach, Walmart also instituted a number of other ways to improve the healthcare outcomes and experiences of their employees. These included (1) using data from public and private insurance programs to create quality/cost reports and steer their employees to physicians with a track record of providing high-quality, cost-effective care; (2) utilizing healthcare assistants to help employees address issues with healthcare billing, find providers, and set up appointments; and (3) expanding low-cost telehealth services to include preventive care, urgent care, behavioral health, and chronic care management.

> The single biggest distinguishing factor about "Centers of Excellence" is not the surgeries they do but the surgeries they *don't* do.

Second to none in this regard, Walmart has a foundational commitment to its customers, a mission that was embedded in the organization by its founder, Sam Walton, who was clearly a 'beyond the walls' thinker and leader. Sam had a belief that was divergent from other mainstream retailers. His vision was for every American and American family to be able to afford quality goods and obtain them

---

124 Personal communication with Walmart executives, 2018–2019.

through respectful service. He and his company fought hard to make that a reality. When accepting the Presidential Medal of Freedom from George H. W. Bush in 1992, Sam said, "If we work together, we'll lower the cost of living for everyone … we'll give the world an opportunity to see what it's like to save and have a better life."

I have to take my hat off to Walmart for its leadership in identifying and analyzing how to deliver the best and most affordable healthcare to its employees and extending that same approach to its customers. It's these principles that form the foundation for much of the work Walmart is doing today in constructing its healthcare ecosystem.

CVS Health

CVS, of course, began as a retail chain of pharmacies. Today it is so much more. Its strategy—to touch every step in the healthcare journey—likely had its roots back in 2018, when CVS completed its acquisition of Aetna in what was a transformative moment for the industry. In 2022 CVS Health spent $8 billion acquiring Signify Health, a leader in health risk assessments, value-based care, and provider enablement. Signify already had in place a network of more than ten thousand clinicians across all fifty states, a nationwide value-based provider network, combined with proprietary analytics and supporting technology platforms.

The financial and clinical benefits that Signify Health brings to CVS include (1) revenue generation from home-based healthcare, (2) more optimal coding and billing that generates multiples on Medicare Advantage payments, (3) the ability to reduce medical expenditures through proactive real-time prevention in patients' homes, and (4) the ability to perform well on quality and experience metrics, leading to higher payment and improved care outcomes. In addition, CVS is developing other internal capabilities, including a post-hospital discharge transitions care service.

Lynch has also announced her intentions to expand CVS Health's services into primary care and more specifically into Medicare Advantage–based senior care. To that end, CVS disclosed plans to acquire primary care company Oak Street Health in February 2023 and completed the $10.6 billion transaction three months later in May 2023. Oak Street Health's primary focus is Medicare Advantage, and they bring nearly 170 clinics in 21 states to CVS, with plans to expand to over 300 clinics by 2026. Under the deal, Oak Street will continue to operate as a multi-payer primary care provider within CVS Health.[125] A press release and statement by Lynch in February 2023 clearly articulated CVS Health's vertical strategy and its desire to become a leading national provider of primary care, "Combining Oak Street Health's platform with CVS Health's unmatched reach will create the premier value-based primary care solution… Enhancing our value-based offerings is core to our strategy as we continue to redefine how people access and experience care that is more affordable, convenient, and connected." Lynch believes CVS has an advantage over some of the other titans because the company has built years of trust with healthcare consumers and continues to do so. Along these lines, she recently stated, "What we did in the pandemic to vaccinate America has really allowed us as a company to earn the right to be in health care."[126]

---

125 Rebecca Pifer, "CVS Closes $10.6B Oak Street Health Buy," healthcaredive.com, May 2, 2023, https://www.healthcaredive.com/news/cvs-closes-oak-street-health-buy/649177/.

126 Lauren Berryman, "Walgreens Eyes Health Tech Acquisition as It Expands Health-care Unit," *Modern Healthcare*, October 13, 2022, https://www.modernhealthcare.com/finance/walgreens-ceo-next-acquisition-may-be-tech-company.

Walgreens

Walgreens, like CVS, is another retail pharmacy chain that is reinventing itself as a healthcare provider and expanding beyond its traditional role through acquisitions. Walgreens fully acquired CareCentrix, a home-based health platform, in 2021 and also invested $5.2 billion in VillageMD that same year for a majority ownership stake. In 2022 VillageMD acquired Summit Health-CityMD, a leading provider of primary, specialty, and urgent care, for close to $9 billion. It's interesting to note that Summit had acquired CityMD (a premier urgent care chain in greater NYC and New Jersey). The humorous but apt metaphor that comes to mind here is that of the matryoshka Russian nesting dolls that stack within one another. Summit, a large multi-specialty provider group, acquired CityMD, a game-changing urgent care chain. VillageMD, a national MA-based PCP, acquired Summit. And finally, the big doll, Walgreens, acquired VillageMD.

The 'nesting doll' strategy—similar to the other titans—is to construct a continuum-of-care ecosystem. But this isn't children playing with dolls. This strategy and these acquisitions are beginning to pay off big for Walgreens. In 2022 VillageMD nearly doubled the number of its clinics to 403, with plans to open 1,000 clinics colocated with Walgreens stores by 2027. VillageMD, Shields, and CareCentrix collectively brought in more than $1.6 billion in revenue in the second quarter of 2023—up from $527 million in sales one year earlier. CEO Rosalind Brewer called it a "landmark quarter," and John Driscoll, president of Walgreens's US healthcare segment, stated, "What we're seeing is the opportunity to drive more cost and growth synergies off of a multi-threat set of assets that we think can be very impactful part as we concentrate market power with more service offerings in specific markets."[127]

SUMMING UP THE GAME PLAN

At the risk of oversimplifying it, the game plan these titans are following can be distilled into the following three key tenets:

1) Amass enough member clients and capitated risk to generate significant revenue, which also enhances market power. Gathering a large client base facilitates negotiating power when the disruptor goes to make deals with suppliers like hospital systems or with customers like self-insured employees. The size of the customer base also provides the opportunity to spread out the cost of new and expensive technologies or expertise.

2) Own and control the capabilities that can have an impact on reducing unnecessary and avoidable medical costs while optimizing revenue. This includes optimizing coding, billing, and the risk adjustment multiplier and optimizing quality and experience scores leading to enhanced revenue. The analytics capability is likely to become a game changer as AI-enabled technology advances. It's critical in identifying patients who are at higher risk for medical care and higher medical costs and even more impactful in proactively identifying patients who are likely to become high risk and therefore high cost.

3) Stay out of the brick-and-mortar hospital game. Hospitals have a tremendous fixed-cost component. In fact, the single largest cost factor in healthcare is hospitalizations, at 31 percent. If you add in the cost of physicians who deliver care in the hospital, that number

---

127 Caroline Hudson, "Walgreens Bets Big on VillageMD as It Expands Healthcare Services," *Modern Healthcare*, March 28, 2023, https://www.modernhealthcare.com/finance/walgreens-villagemd-operating-income-earnings-2nd-quarter-2023.

would be at least five percentage points higher.[128] As the new entrants reduce the costliest part of healthcare utilization, they're also reducing hospital revenue, which creates a quagmire for hospital-based healthcare systems and their revenue model. Regarding the costs of specialty care or surgical care, the titans have options. First, they can modulate the number of specialists they hire to meet their needs rather than employ them and add overutilization costs. Second, they can acquire or contract with ASCs, which are a lower-cost alternative to hospital-based surgical procedures. And third, they can contract with hospital systems for specialty care as well as surgical care—likely in some negotiated, bundled-payment arrangement.

SECTION 3: THE PAYVIDERS

Let's switch gears and focus on the other major category of titans of disruption. I referred to this group earlier as healthcare insurance companies or what we call "payers." But the more accurate label is "payviders"—a combination of payer and provider. The payvider model is a vertically integrated approach where the payer merges with a provider to share both the risk and rewards of managing member care. The payviders we're about to discuss all began as health insurance companies. But just like the retailers, they are expanding into different areas of care delivery in their efforts to gain market share and garner more of the healthcare dollar.

Humana

Humana is less than a third of the size of the UnitedHealthcare Group, the largest health insurer, in terms of revenue. Still, it's at least twice as

---

128 "Trends in Health Care Spending," American Medical Association, March 20, 2023, https://www.ama-assn.org/about/research/trends-health-care-spending.

large as the largest hospital-based healthcare system. Humana is also incredibly forward-thinking, as witnessed by the tremendous investments it has been making in home-based care and senior care.

In 2018 Humana began partnering up with Kindred at Home, one of the largest home-based care companies, which Humana acquired outright for roughly $8 billion in 2021. (They have since sold 60 percent of it back, the part focused on hospice, to a private equity firm.) They also invested $100 million into a partnership with Heal, which provides in-home comprehensive primary care through house calls and one-touch telemedicine. In 2020 they formed a strategic partnership with DispatchHealth, another home-based provider of acute and nonacute medical services and have since invested in that company across three rounds of funding.[129] DispatchHealth has become a hospital-at-home powerhouse but has also expanded its home-based clinical portfolio to the entire continuum of care, including urgent care, emergency care, chronic disease management, and long-term care.

This portfolio of acquisitions and investments serves mostly seniors, which makes clear what market segment Humana is targeting. To punctuate that point, Humana recently announced that it was completely exiting the commercial insurance market.[130] This is a huge strategic move that is consistent with the investments the company has made over the last decade. Today only UnitedHealthcare (at 28

---

129 "DispatchHealth Raises More Than $330 Million to Expand Its Technology-Enabled Ecosystem of High Acuity Care in the Home," Cision PR Newswire, November 23, 2022, https://www.prnewswire.com/news-releases/dispatchhealth-raises-more-than-330-million-to-expand-its-technology-enabled-ecosystem-of-high-acuity-care-in-the-home-301686594.html.

130 "Humana to Exit Employer Group Commercial Medical Products Business," Humana, February 23, 2023, https://press.humana.com/news/news-details/2023/Humana-to-Exit-Employer-Group-Commercial-Medical-Products-Business/.

percent) has higher Medicare Advantage enrollment than Humana, which has 18 percent of the total Medicare Advantage market.[131]

On the clinical side, Humana has invested close to $2 billion in senior care clinics. In a brilliant move, Humana consolidated its senior care clinics and its Kindred at Home services into one *CenterWell* brand. They currently have 220 clinics in 11 states located in the Southeast and Southwest, thereby targeting the largest- and fastest-growing senior populations in the country. Their goal in 2023 is to open an additional 30–35 senior-focused primary care centers across Virginia, North and South Carolina, Tennessee, Kentucky, Texas, Louisiana, Mississippi, Nevada, and Indiana and to continue that pace in the subsequent years.[132] With the company having invested heavily in home health, it's poised to also capture highly profitable diagnoses for patients who otherwise couldn't come for in-person care, as well as accrue all of the other benefits of a home health business line described in section I of this chapter.

To be sure, this alignment of Humana's Medicare Advantage insurance products with its clinical investments in senior care and home-based care capabilities is a highly strategic and intentional tactic—a focused, multiyear, stepwise strategy that its executives and its CEO have been very public about. CEO Bruce Broussard stated in 2020, "We believe the movement of care toward the home will shape the coming decade."[133] Humana has a short, middle, and long game and is on a solid trajectory to becoming a titan of disruption

131 Meredith Freed et al., "Medicare Advantage in 2022: Enrollment Update and Key Trends," Kaiser Family Foundation, August 25, 2022, https://www.kff.org/medicare/issue-brief/medicare-advantage-in-2022-enrollment-update-and-key-trends/.

132 "CenterWell Senior Primary Care 2023 Expansion Plan Includes New Markets of Indiana, Mississippi and Virginia," Humana, November 16, 2022, https://press.humana.com/news/news-details/2022/CenterWell-Senior-Primary-Care-2023-Expansion-Plan-Includes-New-Markets-of-Indiana-Mississippi-and-Virginia/.

133 "Humana's Long-Term Strategy," Oliver Wyman, February 2020, https://www.oliverwyman.com/our-expertise/perspectives/health/2020/sep/humana-s-president-and-ceo-on-healthcare-s-future.html.

in the healthcare industry as well as a dominant, integrated payvider of senior care. There is little doubt that these moves are financially sound and have contributed to Humana's sustained revenue and membership growth. Over the past four years, Humana's individual Medicare Advantage annual growth rate of 10.4 percent has consistently surpassed the industry rate of 9.7 percent. Most recently, the company announced that it had achieved 22 percent year-over-year growth in adjusted earnings per share despite its 60 percent divestiture of Kindred Hospice.[134]

UnitedHealth Group

UnitedHealth Group (UHG) is the largest of the payviders, and it's been flexing its market muscles for some time.

In 2011 UHG formed its Optum subsidiary to handle existing pharmacy, analytics, and care delivery services. In 2017 Optum accounted for 44 percent of UHG's profits. By 2020 it contributed more than 50 percent to UHG's earnings. One of its components, Optum Health, employs or contracts with more than sixty thousand providers, including primary care, medical specialty care, and surgical care. Optum has also made other numerous acquisitions in the healthcare space, such as naviHealth, which provides postacute care management; AbleTo, a virtual behavioral health company; Landmark, one of the giants in home-based care visits (described in chapter 4); and Vivify Health, which specializes in remote monitoring of home patients.

Again, UHG began as an insurance-based company. But now its subsidiaries make more than its foundational business. And UHG's size is staggering. The largest hospital system in the country brings

---

134   "Q4 2022 Humana Inc Earnings Call," Humana, February 1, 2023, https://humana. gcs-web.com/static-files/0df7d740-3c7f-4d2e-90d9-5cbde222db17.

in roughly $30 billion in annual revenue, while Optum Rx, UHG's pharmacy benefits management company, alone is in the $90 to $100 billion annual revenue range![135]

UHG also has OptumInsight, which may be one of the most advanced healthcare analytics companies in the country. OptumInsight has recently acquired another insurance analytics business, Change Healthcare. The publicly shared concern among other payers as well as hospital systems is that Change Healthcare has been working with many other insurance companies, which led to the acquisition being challenged by UHG's competitors and the Federal Trade Commission. Despite challenges, that acquisition closed in October 2022. UHG also acquired divvyDOSE, which is similar to Amazon's PillPack in that they send out prepackaged prescription pills through the mail. The upshot—Optum is generating $324 billion in revenue through at least four completely different lines of businesses, each of which has its own subsidiaries.

UHG's strategy is similar to Humana and the other titans— amass enough patients to become relevant and have power in different markets, take on capitated risk for those patients (primarily through Medicare Advantage), and then own and control the capabilities that can identify inefficiencies (like analytics) and are most able to impact costs (primary care, home-based care, and pharmacy). UHG also seems to be committed to diversification and building up businesses that are profitable in and of themselves. An example is its acquisition of ambulatory surgery centers through Surgical Care Affiliates, now rebranded as SCA Health, a subsidiary of Optum that was acquired in 2017. At the time of this writing, SCA owns approximately 320 ambulatory surgery centers in over 30 states, and close to 12,000

---

135 "UnitedHealth Group Reports 2022 Results," UnitedHealth Group, January 13, 2023, https://www.unitedhealthgroup.com/content/dam/UHG/PDF/investors/2022/UNH-Q4-2022-Release.pdf.

surgeons utilize their facilities. While the surgeons are not employees, there is co-ownership of these ambulatory surgery centers with SCA; therefore, they and partnering health systems share in the profitability.

SECTION 4: TAILWINDS AND HEADWINDS

Tailwinds

SIZE

The titans have some significant tailwinds propelling their ability to disrupt and advance. We mentioned this particular tailwind earlier in the chapter. I've labeled these organizations as titans, in part, because they're massive revenue generators. They have a much greater cushion of capital than the lower revenue/lower margin legacy healthcare systems. This gives them significantly more leverage when it comes to investing in new acquisitions, assets, and capabilities, as well as for growth, R & D, and piloting and testing new programs. They also have a lot more room to make mistakes. For example, Amazon threw in the towel on Amazon Care, its in-house primary care offering, and instead purchased One Medical as its national PCP. This was a move that was highly criticized in the press but one that I saw as brilliantly strategic and bold.

DIVERSIFICATION

The disruptors also have the advantage of a business model that leverages tremendous revenue diversification. For example, in 2021 UHG made $223 billion in revenue from its insurance arm, $91 billion from pharmacy benefits management (PBM), and $12 billion from its analytics and operational services arm. Its provider revenue was $54 billion, far beyond that of any hospital-based healthcare system but still only a fraction of its very large and diversified portfolio. That $54 billion represents less than 15 percent of UHG's entire revenue.

We can run the same analysis for CVS Health. In 2021 that company earned $82 billion in revenue from Aetna, its insurance arm; $100 billion from its retail and healthcare delivery arm; and $153 billion from its PBM. Given that CVS is largely recognized as a retailer, it's surprising to learn that CVS's PBM is, by far, its largest stream of revenue.

HEALTH INSURANCE GIANTS CONTINUING TO DIVERSIFY
Provider, Pharmacy, and Other Services Arms Growing as Fast or Faster than Insurance Segments

Year Over Year Payer Revenue Growth, by Segment
IN BILLIONS ($)

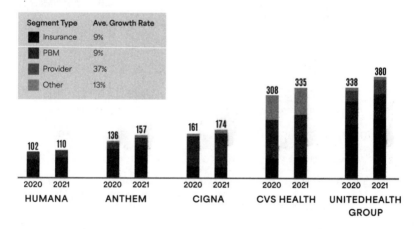

In this graphic from the Gist Healthcare publication, you can see the power of these companies' diversification efforts.[136] That power gives them a profound advantage compared with hospital-based healthcare systems whose major diversifications are real estate, financial investments, and some commercial investments—diversifications all of the titans have as well.

---

136 "Payers Racing to Expand Their Provider Footprints," Gist Healthcare, March 3, 2023, https://gisthealthcare.com/payers-racing-to-expand-their-provider-footprints/.

THE FLYWHEEL EFFECT

The flywheel effect, which we discussed in chapter 7, is the notion of building a set of offerings that create a momentum of consumer awareness, engagement, and utilization.[137] By having a broad but aligned portfolio of related healthcare offerings, these disruptors can create that flywheel effect in a big way. They possess a strong cross-selling advantage, as they have feeders and other channels for revenue generation. Once you're in, say, UHG's system, the company can take you from one of their subsidiaries to another. For example, you're able to get your primary care, your prescription benefits, and your insurance all within UHG's portfolio.

DECADES OF CONSUMER ORIENTATION

These disruptors put a marketing mindset front and center in their business endeavors. They understand customer segmentation—how to identify products and services consumers value, how to identify the size of that addressable market, how to test these potential products and optimize a strong product-market fit, how to design and develop new products and services, how to conduct nationally scaled market rollouts of their products and services, how to do postmarket testing, and how to acquire and retain consumers through marketing. This is not a new set of skills for them, but it is a relatively new set of skills for hospital-based systems.

CONVENIENCE

The disruptors make it a point to provide quick and easy access, making them far more attractive to consumers. Time is important to most people, and it seems that retailers understand that in a way

---

137   Sara Vaezy and Doug Grapski, "Dig This: Why HealthCare Needs a Flywheel," Providence, August 9, 2022, https://blog.providence.org/digital-innovation-content/dig-this-why-healthcare-needs-a-flywheel.

that the traditional healthcare systems have not yet fully grasped. To drive this point home, 50 percent of all Amazon purchases occur in a time frame of fifteen minutes or less, and 28 percent of purchases occur in three minutes or less.[138] Another facet of convenience is the one-stop-shop idea. Customers who visit CVS, Walmart, Walgreens, and Amazon can obtain their healthcare, their medications, and other health-related products and equipment and then shop for nonmedical items such as groceries and household supplies.

CONSUMER BASE

A total of 90 percent of Americans live within ten miles of a Walmart store, resulting in that company serving 140 million US customers weekly. Amazon has over 42 million unique desktop users and over 126 million unique mobile visitors in the United States each month.[139] Over a quarter of prescriptions in the United States are filled at CVS, and nearly half of all Americans are CVS customers, with the typical customer making a trip to CVS every other week.[140] The payviders are mostly national players, so they, too, have a huge customer base to which they can market and sell their products and services. These titans can get a much higher return on their investment in products and services because of the opportunity to spread and scale them nationally, whereas legacy healthcare systems are typically more geographically bounded.

---

138   Daisy Quaker, "Amazon Stats: Growth, Sales, and More," Amazon, March 31, 2022, https://sell.amazon.com/blog/grow-your-business/amazon-stats-growth-and-sales,

139   Quaker, "Amazon Stats: Growth, Sales, and More."

140   Dominick Reuter, "Meet the Typical CVS Shopper: A White, Gen X, College-Educated City Dweller Earning a High Income," *Business Insider*, February 27, 2022, https://www.businessinsider.com/ typical-cvs-shopper-demographic-urban-genx-earning-high-income-2021-9.

BUSINESS MODEL ALIGNMENT AND SYNERGIES

There is greater alignment with their business model, especially those with insurance capabilities. These complementary business lines (of payer and provider) afford them the ability to generate revenue on clinical care, on cost savings, and through insurance administrative fees. It's tough to beat this business model, even for healthcare systems that are in shared-risk or full-risk contracts.

SERVICE SOLUTIONS

Many of the titans own service solutions, such as data analytics, care management services, back-office services, technology services, and cloud computing services, that are utilized by healthcare systems and even their insurance competitors. Historically, hospital-based companies have not offered these types of services, although that's beginning to change.

LESS INFRASTRUCTURE EXPENSE

Because the titans have not yet invested in costly hospital infrastructure, they don't have those expenses to weigh them down. I suspect that they will be utilizing the hospital-at-home approach, given its lower total costs (20 to 40 percent less) compared with brick-and-mortar hospitals.[141] They will likely rely on contracts with the highest-quality surgeons and medical interventionalists, trading guaranteed volume for significant reductions in price, similar to Amazon and Walmart today, and they are already partnering with hospital-at-home vendors such as DispatchHealth and Medically Home. I believe we're going to see them following Optum's lead in partnering with and

---

141 Haley Brider, "Home Hospital Model Reduces Costs by 38%, Study Says," *Harvard Gazette*, December 16, 2019, https://news.harvard.edu/gazette/story/2019/12/home-hospital-model-reduces-costs-by-38-improves-care; Aditya Achanta and David Velasquez, "Hospital at Home: Paying for What It's Worth," *American Journal of Managed Care* 27, no. 9 (2021): 369–371, https://doi.org/10.37765/ajmc.2021.88739.

acquiring ASCs, another lower-cost option versus the hospital-based surgical suites.

ANALYTIC CAPABILITIES

Finally, these entities have been collecting, analyzing, and acting on consumer and cost data for decades. Consumer analytics is their lifeblood. It is how they can take insurance risk on healthcare. These are powerhouses of analytic capability that exceed the abilities of hospital-based systems.

TAILWINDS FOR THE TITANS OF DISRUPTION

- Size
- Business model/revenue diversification
- The flywheel effect
- Decades of consumer orientation
- Convenience
- Consumer base
- Business model alignment and synergies
- Service solutions
- Less infrastructure expense
- Analytic capabilities

Headwinds

A NATIONAL ORIENTATION SPREAD THIN

Yes, these are huge companies with a national presence. However, their footprint in any specific region could still be relatively small.

This doesn't mean they can't win big. It just means that they may not be able to dominate a particular market. From a competitive perspective, this sounds like good news for hospital systems. The bad news for hospital systems is that we're not talking about one titan. We're talking about *all* of them.

RELATIVE LACK OF PUBLIC TRUST

Consumers certainly trust these retailers in terms of shopping for goods and prescriptions or getting a flu shot. However, if you or a family member are sick with something beyond a mild cold or a blood pressure check, are you going to trust your care to CVS Health or Amazon? That's a question that remains to be answered. One thing is clear: people are more likely to trust their PCP when they make their healthcare decisions. CVS recently released a study in which 59 percent of consumers stated that their PCP was their most trusted healthcare provider, and 27 percent of consumers said that trust had increased since the pandemic.[142] Will consumers trust a PCP who has CVS, Amazon, or Walmart on their prescription pad? A recent study from Wolters Kluwer Health provides some clues. The study reported that 61 percent of consumers believed their PCP would come from retail settings in the next five years, but that number dropped to 43 percent for baby boomers, who actually have the most healthcare needs today.[143] So it's still unclear if healthcare consumers will readily adopt retail-driven primary care in large numbers. The advantage hospital systems and their vast network of doctors have is that they

---

142 "2022 Health Care Insights Study," CVS Health, 2022, https://www.cvshealth.com/content/dam/enterprise/cvs-enterprise/pdfs/cvs-health-care-insights-study-2022-report-executive-summary.pdf.

143 "U.S. Survey Signals Big Shifts in Primary Care to Pharmacy and Clinic Settings as Consumers Seek Lower Medication and Healthcare Costs," Wolters Kluwer, December 7, 2022, https://www.wolterskluwer.com/en/news/us-survey-signals-big-shifts-in-primary-care-to-pharmacy-and-clinic-settings.

are community based and have conceivably developed trust within their communities. We'll return to this issue of trust in chapter 9.

A REGULATED ENVIRONMENT

Healthcare, as opposed to normal retail sales, is a highly regulated and complex environment. It takes time and expertise to work within that system, and many of these companies are still at the beginning of their expansion into healthcare. They have a steep learning curve ahead of them. On the other hand, most are utilizing healthcare veterans who can guide them through regulatory and other hoops.

LOWER PROFITABILITY

The disruptors could discover that healthcare provision may not be as profitable as their other revenue streams. The healthcare market is witnessing downward pressures on revenue and increases in labor and supply costs.[144] CMS and HHS are continuing to actively implement policies and rules to reduce healthcare costs, particularly in Medicare Advantage, which makes up approximately half of all Medicare enrollees. One recent example is a Medicare Advantage audit rule that caused an uproar in the healthcare insurance industry.[145] Another very recent shock wave in the industry was caused by proposed CMS rules to remove approximately two thousand diagnostic codes from the risk adjustment model, which will lower payments to insurers by

---

144 Laura Dyrda, "What Hospitals Can Expect from Labor Costs in 2023," Becker's Healthcare, January 25, 2023, https://www.beckershospitalreview.com/finance/what-hospitals-can-expect-from-labor-costs-in-2023.html.

145 Reed Abelson and Margo Sanger-Katz, "New Medicare Rule Aims to Take Back $4.7 Billion from Insurers," New York Times, January 30, 2023, https://www.nytimes.com/2023/01/30/upshot/medicare-overbilling-biden-rule.html.

billions of dollars per year.[146, 147] And another example is the Inflation Reduction Act that President Biden signed in August 2020, which allows Medicare to negotiate lower prescription drug prices, caps the cost of insulin, makes vaccines free to Medicare beneficiaries, and requires pharmaceutical companies to pay rebates if they raise drug prices faster than inflation.[148, 149] These and other revenue pressures are sure to come, as the overall costs of healthcare are untenable for the majority of Americans and unsustainable for governmental and commercial payers. On the other hand, if these titans can garner even 20 percent of a $4 trillion American healthcare industry, that would more than double the revenue for even the largest retailer.[150]

CHALLENGE OF INTEGRATION

These disruptors are large, and so far, I've positioned that quality as a positive. But there's a shadow side to acquisitions and partnerships. It can be unwieldy to integrate and coordinate all these assets and have them work together, especially within the complexities of the healthcare regulatory environment. For anyone that's been involved in any sort of merger, you understand all too well that it's one thing to acquire or merge and something completely different to integrate. For example, Teladoc

---

146   Reed Abelson and Margo Sanger-Katz, "Medicare Delays a Full Crackdown on Private Health Plans," *New York Times*, March 31, 2023, https://www.nytimes.com/2023/03/31/health/medicare-overbilling-insurance.html.

147   Victoria Bailey, "Stakeholder Groups Oppose Medicare Advantage Risk Adjustment Changes," *Health Payer Intelligence*, March 16, 2023, https://healthpayerintelligence.com/news/stakeholder-groups-oppose-medicare-advantage-risk-adjustment-changes.

148   "The Inflation Reduction Act Lowers Health Care Costs for Millions of Americans," Centers for Medicare & Medicaid Services, October 5, 2022, https://www.cms.gov/newsroom/fact-sheets/inflation-reduction-act-lowers-health-care-costs-millions-americans.

149   Paula Span, "Medicare Begins to Rein in Drug Costs for Older Americans," *New York Times*, January 14, 2023, https://www.nytimes.com/2023/01/14/health/medicare-drug-prices.html.

150   "Historical," Centers for Medicare & Medicaid Services, accessed April 19, 2023, https://www.cms.gov/research-statistics-data-and-systems/statistics-trends-and-reports/nationalhealthexpenddata/nationalhealthaccountshistorical.

recently recorded a $6.6 billion impairment charge on Livongo, the digital health company it acquired in late 2020 for $18.5 billion. Teladoc executives stated that the drop in value resulted from poor timing as more Americans returned to in-person care in 2021 that lowered demand for virtual healthcare solutions. But others point to poor execution of the deal on multiple levels—from cultural and operational integration misjudgments to business development errors. Additionally, within a year of the deal, all but one of Livongo's management team had departed, suggesting another major misstep on Teladoc's part. Given all of that, the company has struggled to meet performance metrics. It also failed to integrate everything into a single consumer app until early 2023, over two years after the deal closed. Finally, Teladoc lost Cigna as a client. The Livongo acquisition demonstrates that what may make sense on paper does not always come to fruition, if it cannot be executed effectively.[151]

HEADWINDS FOR THE TITANS OF DISRUPTION

- A national orientation spread thin
- (Relative) Lack of public trust
- A regulated environment
- Lower profitability
- Challenges of integration

---

151 Rebecca Pifer, "Teladoc Records $6.6B Impairment Charge on Livongo Acquisition, Spurring Record Net Loss," Healthcare Dive, April 27, 2022, https://www.healthcaredive.com/news/teladoc-records-66b-impairment-charge-on-livongo-acquisition-spurring-re/622793/; Brock Turner, "Teladoc Health Ties Up Livongo Merger with New App," *Digital Health Modern Healthcare*, January 6, 2023, https://digitalhealth.modernhealthcare.com/mergers-acquisitions-ma/teladoc-health-ties-up-livongo-merger-new-app.

OTHER DISRUPTORS THAT SHOULD BE CONSIDERED

A major set of disruptions will emerge from the employer space, keeping in mind that employers pay for over 40 percent of the health-care bills in the United States. Since 1999 average premiums for employer-sponsored insurance have risen over 250 percent to $7,739 for an individual and $22,221 for a family.[152] These increases have occurred despite employees taking on more of the burden in paying for care through higher deductibles, coinsurance, and co-pays.[153] One employer-based strategy to contain these cost pressures is to drop out of conventional insurance plans and self-insure their own healthcare. Another strategy is direct-to-employer contracting, which we'll touch upon in chapter 9.[154]

Another major stakeholder, which we mentioned a couple of pages back, is the federal government. The CMS, the Centers for Medicare & Medicaid Services, as well as its Center for Medicare & Medicaid Innovation, has a mandate to develop and test new healthcare payment and service delivery models and to better align payment systems with patient-centered practices. CMS is the payer for Medicare and, in part, for Medicaid services, comprising over 30 percent of healthcare payments in the United States. They've had, and will continue to have, a significant impact in advancing value-based payment, especially with their recent "strategy refresh."[155] CMS also

---

152 "2021 Employer Health Benefits Survey—Section 1: Cost of Health Insurance," Kaiser Family Foundation, November 10, 2021, https://www.kff.org/report-section/ehbs-2021-section-1-cost-of-health-insurance/.

153 "2021 Employer Health Benefits Survey—Section 7: Employee Cost Sharing," Kaiser Family Foundation, November 10, 2021, https://www.kff.org/report-section/ehbs-2021-section-7-employee-cost-sharing/.

154 "2021 Employer Health Benefits Survey—Section 10: Plan Funding," Kaiser Family Foundation, November 10, 2021, https://www.kff.org/report-section/ehbs-2021-section-10-plan-funding/.

155 "Innovation Center Strategy Refresh," Centers for Medicare & Medicaid Services, 2021, https://innovation.cms.gov/strategic-direction-whitepaper.

creates the payment policies for Medicare Advantage, which has a huge ripple effect in the market, given that Medicare Advantage is currently 50 percent of all Medicare payments and projected to cover over 60 percent of all Medicare enrollees by 2030.[156] One additional influence CMS possesses is that commercial payers often follow the lead that CMS sets. The federal government will become an even greater market force as it attempts to rein in costs in the face of the looming insolvency of the Medicare Trust Fund, projected to run out of money in 2028.[157]

Another major market disruption is the entrance of VC and private equity into the healthcare industry. Over the past few years, we've seen a rapid rise in the tens of billions of dollars being invested each year by VC. In the last ten years, private equity has invested $1 trillion in nearly eight thousand healthcare transactions.[158] The topic is a hot one for sure, as more and more provider groups are being acquired by or partnering with these entities and as the titans also partner with VC firms in their market-shifting acquisitions and partnerships. The VC buying spree in healthcare began in higher margin specialty groups such as radiology and anesthesiology. But now we're seeing PCP groups being acquired by VCs, especially those engaged in Medicare Advantage contracting.

We also need to open our awareness to internationally based disruptors. In countries such as India, entrepreneurial healthcare leaders are attempting to solve complexities in that nation's healthcare system

156 Michael McWilliams, "Don't Look Up? Medicare Advantage's Trajectory and the Future of Medicare," *Health Affairs*, March 24, 2022, https://www.healthaffairs.org/do/10.1377/forefront.20220323.773602/.

157 Juliette Cubanski and Tricia Neuman, "FAQs on Medicare Financing and Trust Fund," Kaiser Family Foundation, June 17, 2022, https://www.kff.org/medicare/issue-brief/faqs-on-medicare-financing-and-trust-fund-solvency/.

158 Fred Schulte, "Sick Profit: Investigating Private Equity's Stealthy Takeover of Health Care across Cities and Specialties," *Kaiser Health News*, November 14, 2022, https://khn.org/news/article/private-equity-takeover-health-care-cities-specialties/.

that may rival, if not surpass, our own. And entrepreneurial hotbed countries such as Israel, the so-called "start-up nation," are creating a multitude of technologic enablements to transform care.[159]

Legacy providers and hospital-based systems are indeed threatened by what the titans of disruption are doing. But this disruption might not be all bad for them, as it may create opportunities for collaborations and partnerships. More importantly, it may create a better healthcare system for patients, providers, and the actual payers of healthcare, the American public. In the next chapter, we'll build upon the generative aspects of the disruption by discussing what hospital-based healthcare systems can and are doing to join in and lead the movement to advance healthcare beyond the walls of its current limitations.

---

159 Dan Senior and Paul Singer, *Start-Up Nation: The Story of Israel's Economic Miracle* (New York: Twelve, 2011).

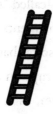

CHAPTER 9

FROM DISRUPTED TO DISRUPTOR: THE POWER OF PARTNERSHIPS

When we set out several years ago ... to transform the healthcare system, we knew we could never do it alone. No one company could "disrupt" healthcare; it would require the creation of an ecosystem of partners.

–Daryl Tol, partner, Health Assurance Ecosystem, General Catalyst

A fter that last chapter, you may be thinking that the game is over, and it's inevitable that these titans of disruption will dominate our national healthcare ecosystem. But following up on the reference to Greek mythology introduced in chapter 8, it's only fair to share the balance of the story—without any intention of foreshadowing. As the myth goes, the Titans were eventually overthrown by the Olympian gods, with Zeus leading the insurrection in a ten-year war known as the Titanomachy. This book is clearly not a work of fictional drama, and it's not based on mythology. The titans we're talking about here are not deities but corporations. And as we touched upon toward the end of the last chapter, they are subject to the same market forces and competitive pressures as any other stakeholder in the healthcare industry. Picking up on that, let's do one more quick reality check on the history of healthcare titans and then explore the advantages and opportunities available to the hospital-based healthcare systems.

Most of us have already forgotten *Haven*, the healthcare partnership formed by Amazon, Berkshire Hathaway, and JPMorgan. Jeff Bezos, founder and CEO of Amazon; Warren Buffett, the oracle from Omaha; and James Dimon, CEO extraordinaire—leaders of the three largest employers in America—banded together to create a new healthcare ecosystem targeted at employees. They hired the best and brightest leaders from across the nation. They had the right idea and all the right ingredients. Experts and pundits predicted that their endeavor was going to redefine American healthcare and disrupt the industry.[160] The behemoth called Haven made its grand entrance onto the national stage in January 2018 and meekly exited the stage just three years later, going from fanfare to fizzle without any fury.[161] It's a cautionary tale in the American healthcare industry.[162] As we touched upon toward the end of chapter 8, there is a wow factor when titans align in multibillion-dollar M&As. But these M&As take years of integration that involve the complex assimilation of things such as

160   Nick Wingfield, Katie Thomas, and Reed Abelson, "Amazon, Berkshire Hathaway and JPMorgan Team Up to Try to Disrupt Health Care," *New York Times*, January 30, 2018, https://www.nytimes.com/2018/01/30/technology/amazon-berkshire-hathaway-jpmorgan-health-care.html.

161   Emily Flitter and Karen Weise, "Amazon, Berkshire and JPMorgan Will End Joint Health Care Venture," *New York Times*, January 4, 2021, https://www.nytimes.com/2021/01/04/business/haven-amazon-berkshire-hathaway-jpmorgan.html.

162   John Toussaint, "Why Haven Healthcare Failed," *Harvard Business Review*, January 6, 2021, https://hbr.org/2021/01/why-haven-healthcare-failed.

strategy, operations, technology, policies, and culture. Titanic deals may be made by the gods, but the devil is in the details.

HOSPITAL SYSTEMS HAVE SOME UNIQUE ADVANTAGES

Despite their numerous advantages, the titans of disruption will have to overcome some substantial challenges, such as gaining and maintaining the trust of the American public, which we touched upon in chapter 8. Hospitals and providers have a clear advantage here. When I speak to leadership at healthcare systems across the country, I refer to trust as one of their "superpowers." Hospital-based health-

> Titanic deals may be made by the gods, but the devil is in the details.

care systems, and their employed and affiliated provider groups, are trusted brands in their communities. The corollary is that hospital systems have a strong customer base. It's much harder to pull established customers away from their trusted brands than it is to attract a customer who has no or little brand allegiance. The hospital-based systems have a solid brand, and they also have the primary and specialty care provider channels to attract and retain customers.

Another superpower belonging to hospital-based systems is their network of integrated care. Integrated care delivery in our legacy systems may be far from ideal, but they're way ahead of the retailers and even the payviders who are still carving out segments of the continuum and attempting to master those.

Finally, hospital-based systems have spent decades developing expertise in managing regulatory, operational, and quality hurdles. This may not sound like a superpower, but it's the difference between playing in the game or sitting on the bench, and more importantly, it's a seal of safety for patient care.

The table below contains a list of what I'm labeling "Hospital System 'Super-Powers' and 'Secret Sauces'"—the market advantages and opportunities that hospital-based systems possess. It's a short-hand checklist distilled from this chapter and previous ones.

HOSPITAL SYSTEM "SUPER-POWERS" AND "SECRET SAUCES"

SUPER-POWERS
- Presence (patients, trusting relationships, large community employer and stakeholder)
- People (operational/clinical knowledge and expertise)
- Platform (a platform business model and a convening integrated system of care)

SECRET SAUCES
- Consolidation (horizontal mergers and acquisitions)
- Collaboration (vertical mergers and partnerships, co-opetition ...)
- Care model transformation (segmentation, customization and engagement, digitalization, virtualization, data-ization ...)

The nomenclature is obviously metaphorical and the two categories have some overlap. I think of "super-powers" as innate assets and capabilities that are an internal part of the organizational infrastructure; whereas "secret sauces" are largely external-facing strategic initiatives and tactics that have been or can be developed. The point is that hospital-based systems have to lean into and leverage their "super-powers," and continue to perfect, advance, and scale their "secret sauces." The corollary is that if they don't, they can easily lose or cede them.

The reality is that other existing and emerging stakeholders can develop these superpowers and secret sauces as well—due, in part, to regulatory changes and shifts in market forces and dynamics. Merely possessing them does not guarantee success. For example, customer loyalty in healthcare is malleable and not as strong as it used to be, especially if lower-cost and more convenient choices become available, as is the titans' ambition. Trust in new alternatives can be built, especially when most Americans simply don't have the time, money, or tolerance to deal with a system that isn't going to adapt to their evolving needs. There is a well-worn quote among the leadership literati—"What got you here won't get you there"—taken from a book by the same name, by Marshall Goldsmith.[163] There is no future for those who insist on staying behind the walls. Hospital-based healthcare systems can and must get beyond the walls if they are to thrive in the future of American healthcare.

So how can legacy healthcare systems compete? And might they eventually rally to become the disruptor rather than the disrupted?

THREE STRATEGIC DOMAINS

There are a number of strategies and tactics legacy healthcare systems can and are taking to remain competitive. The present wisdom is that

---

163 Marshall Goldsmith, *What Got You Here Won't Get You There* (New York: Hachette Books, 2007).

there are three general domains of strategy: (1) running the business—improving efficiency and productivity, as well as quality, safety, reliability, and customer experience; (2) expanding the business—doing more of the same but in a bigger way or expanding into proximal business lines; and (3) growing new businesses—generating new revenue streams.

The third domain isn't about doing the same things more efficiently or even more effectively. It's about doing *different* things that approach effectiveness and efficiency in novel ways.[164,165]

As I write this, there are tremendous financial pressures on hospital-based systems. So the first strategic domain is critical—to improve efficiencies and reduce costs, including removing any unnecessary or duplicative expenditures. The second domain, business expansion, is also critical, and an example is increasing the number of hospital beds, either within existing hospitals (as in new wings or floors) or by building or acquiring hospitals. Another dominant second-domain strategy is the merging of large hospital systems. And while the number of hospital mergers has decreased in recent years, the average size of mergers has grown. In 2021 and 2022, 15 to 16 percent of all hospital mergers included a smaller entity that had at least $1 billion in revenue compared with only 9 percent in 2017, and 30 percent had at least $500 million in revenue. In 2022 the average size of the smaller entity in a hospital merger was a record $852 million in revenue, over twice as large as the average size over the previous ten years.[166] It is almost certain that hospital mergers will continue to be

---

164 Bansi Nagji and Geoff Tuff, "Managing Your Innovation Portfolio," *Harvard Business Review*, May 2012, https://hbr.org/2012/05/managing-your-innovation-portfolio.

165 Millan Alvarez-Miranda and Michael Watkins, "How New CEOs Can Balance Strategy and Execution," *Harvard Business Review*, July 2021, https://hbr.org/2021/07/how-new-ceos-can-balance-strategy-and-execution.

166 "2022 M&A in Review: Regaining Momentum," KaufmanHall, January 12, 2023, https://www.kaufmanhall.com/insights/research-report/2022-ma-review-regaining-momentum.

a mainstay strategy, and it's likely to pick up steam over the next few years as small- and medium-sized hospital systems find it too challenging to remain independently viable entities. It was recently reported that eight hospitals lapsed on their bond payments in Q1 2023, and there is a strong sentiment in the market that more hospitals will falter financially.[167, 168] And while there are numerous critiques about hospital megamergers, the logic is straightforward. Larger size allows for greater combined revenue and absolute margin. These mergers also create the potential for economies of scale in administrative services and even in some clinical service lines, allowing for lower costs and therefore greater margins. As well, there is the significant benefit of negotiating power with payers and suppliers.

The first and second strategic domains are critically important, especially under the current market pressures hospital-based systems are facing. But one lesson from the business world is that for successful companies to maintain their success, they must have a foothold in *all three* strategic domains. If you take your eye off the first two domains, you risk going out of business in the short or medium run. If you take your eye off the third domain, you risk not having a business in the long run. While the majority of resources, capital, and energy are expended on domains one and two, it's the third domain that delivers, by far, the highest return on investment.

For that reason, the focus of this chapter is largely on this third strategic domain involving the generating of new businesses and new revenue streams; more specifically, we'll hone in on one strategy—vertical partnerships—that I see as having the greatest potential positive impact.

---

167 Andrew Cass, "Hospitals See Most 1st-Quarter Defaults Since 2011," Becker's Health-care, April 3, 2023, https://www.beckershospitalreview.com/finance/hospitals-see-most-1st-quarter-defaults-since-2011.html.

168 Lauren Coleman-Lochner, "Hospitals Hit Troubling Milestone in Most 1Q Defaults Since 2011," *Bloomberg*, March 31, 2023.

HOSPITAL-BASED SYSTEMS AND VERTICAL PARTNERSHIPS

As we discovered in the previous chapter, there are numerous examples of vertical partnerships that disruptive titans have engaged in over the past few years, creating great strategic advantage. In contrast, the legacy health systems have relied much more on horizontal mergers. One vulnerability of horizontal partnerships is that all their operating revenue is dependent on a limited portfolio of revenue streams. Why wouldn't legacy hospital-based healthcare systems take a lesson from the titans' playbook? Well, as a matter of fact, that's exactly what they are doing.

Let's begin with one particularly novel type of vertical partnership—the rapidly emerging partnerships between hospital systems and VC firms. A confluence of factors have contributed to this partnership being mutually beneficial. There are tremendous pockets of intellectual property within healthcare systems, including ideas from providers; new programs, services, and technologies emerging from internal innovation divisions; and of course, discoveries being made through formal research. The missing piece here has been the systematic development, commercialization, and scaling of these ideas.

To put it plainly, new product development has not been a core focus for hospitals. That's where the VC firms come into play. These firms are constantly looking for new, profitable, and scalable opportunities to invest in. They provide the funding as well as expert guidance to take a new product to market. Some of the specific value VC firms bring to bear is that they identify and vet new potential offerings, provide early-stage funding to design and develop those ideas into prototypes, vet those prototypes for market desirability, provide further rounds of funding to continue the iterative design and development into consumer-grade products and services, recruit executives to lead a spin-off company with go-to-market capabilities, and manage all of that in partnership with the hospital-based healthcare system.

New product development represents a huge opportunity for hospital-based systems to take nascent products and services to market, to extend beyond their local market, to create new sources of margin-generating revenue, and to serve their mission by having a positive impact on a far greater number of people. To take advantage of this opportunity, hospital systems must (1) invest internally in third domain strategies, expertise, and resources; (2) partner vertically with VC firms and other innovation accelerators; and (3) spin off these products and services into autonomous subsidiary companies.

This last point is the fundamental lesson that renowned Harvard Business School professor Clay Christensen wrote about in *The Innovator's Dilemma*. The way out of the dilemma, and the way for an emerging business line to succeed, is to spin it off as a separate entity. VC partnerships enable this by facilitating the creation of separate subsidiary entities with autonomous leadership, governance, and funding. They provide independent funding to create an independent business line without detracting or distracting from the healthcare system's primary business and core revenue streams. That external funding is needed now, more than ever, as postpandemic revenue and cost challenges plague hospital systems in what could be described as a financial crisis. It also makes perfect sense for these systems to diversify their business lines and provide some stability when primary sources of revenue experience shortfalls.

HOSPITAL-BASED SYSTEMS AND VENTURE CAPITAL PARTNERSHIPS

In October 2022 Allina Health, a hospital-based healthcare system located in Minnesota, announced that it was creating a "spin-out start-up" designed to enable other healthcare systems to jump-start their own hospital-at-home and skilled-nursing-facility-at-home programs. The stated goal was to commercialize Allina Health's home-based care programs and expand into three or four markets outside of the state within one year and then into fifteen additional markets within four years. Their product portfolio is comprehensive and well thought out. It includes an AI-enabled analytics platform to identify ideal patients who would benefit from these services, 24/7 home-based monitoring of patients' vital signs facilitated by a communications hub, a virtual connection to clinicians via video visits, support for payer contracting and supply chain management, support with local caregiver visit coordination, mobile lab and imaging support, and even access to the gig economy part-time workforce. But—and this is the point—they're not attempting to go it alone. The press release indicated that Flare Capital, the VC firm funding and coleading the vertical partnership, was going to raise $20 million in a series A round of funding to resource the start-up.

At about the same time as the Allina/Flare Capital partnership was made public, there was another similar announcement. This one came from a world-class academic medical center specializing in musculoskeletal health—the Hospital for Special Surgery (HSS) located in Manhattan, New York. HSS announced the launch of "RightMove Powered by HSS," an independent for-profit company whose mission is to make high-quality virtual physical therapy available to all Americans. Again, Flare Capital coled a $21 million series A round of funding to support this start-up. This is an absolutely brilliant example of unleashing value from a vertical partnership between a hospital system and a VC firm—taking a homegrown and geographically limited service and making it available to people across the country. The HSS press release pointed out that half of US adults experience musculoskeletal issues, leading to an annual national health expenditure of over $380 billion.[169] Additionally, access to high-quality physical therapy has been shown to reduce unnecessary surgeries, injections, emergency room visits, and imaging studies, leading to better outcomes and lower costs for patients, for payers, and for employers. If there is a win-win-win strategy, this is it. Just imagine what value could be created if other hospital-based systems began to emulate HSS's third domain, 'beyond the walls' strategy. Here are a few important takeaways:

1. In both the Allina and HSS example, they are not disrupting their core business. Instead, they are creating a significant market disruption. These are prime examples of the disrupted becoming the disruptor.

2. They did not attempt to expand the business model within the confines of the organization. Instead, they realized that, in order to thrive and scale this new revenue stream, they would have to form a separate subsidiary business with independent funding and financials, governance and leadership, and operations. They avoided the slog of attempting to launch this from within, fighting an uphill battle against the dominance of their well-established, high-margin core business lines.

---

169   Annie Burky, "Hospital for Special Surgery Scores $21M to Spin Off Virtual Physical Therapy Platform," *Fierce Healthcare*, October 26, 2022, https://www.fiercehealthcare.com/telehealth/hospital-special-surgery-scored-21m-series-funding-spin-virtual-physical-therapy.

3. Flare Capital is not only funding these "spin-off start-ups," but it's also bringing its business-building expertise, which includes finding highly competent senior executives to lead and manage these new businesses. They're also minimizing the risks and maximizing the funding capital by bringing other VC firms on board. In the case of RightMove, Flare Capital has recruited a veteran retail healthcare executive, Marcus Osborne, of Walmart fame to be the CEO of this new venture. And Frist Cressey Ventures and Greycroft, two respected VC firms, have joined as investment partners.

4. These vertical partnerships are not to be confused with traditional consulting relationships. Flare Capital is not charging a consulting fee. They're bringing capital *into* the relationship and de-risking the initiative for the hospital system. This point may sound trivial to those outside of healthcare, but it's pivotal. The funding required to launch such ventures is significant, even for large healthcare systems. A $21 million request for the first round of funding for a new business line is no small ask, especially in revenue-constrained times.

5. The stated purpose of both start-ups is to scale broadly. Allina is planning to expand to fifteen markets outside of Minnesota within four years. HSS is planning to scale nationally, and I suspect they'll be scaling internationally as well. It's unlikely that this level of scaling would have happened without the company being spun off.

Finally, keep in mind that none of this would have been likely, or even possible, if Allina and HSS hadn't partnered with a VC firm. This vertical partnership creates a solution where everyone benefits.

These partnerships extend beyond the VC firm just funding a product or service. The recent partnership between Bassett Healthcare Network in New York State and Andreessen Horowitz (also known as a16z) is a good example. In this instance, Bassett will be leveraging the capabilities of the VC firm's portfolio of digital health companies to solve the challenges and systemic inequities in delivering care to patients living in rural areas. A quote from one of their press releases articulates the vision: "The two organizations share a common vision of broadly reimagining how digital health solutions and processes at scale may transform these valued yet significantly under-resourced healthcare delivery networks." The CEO and president of Bassett, Dr. Tommy Ibrahim, comments, "Partnering with a16z will significantly improve our access to the most innovative digital health technologies and, more broadly, allow us to together truly understand how rural health systems can implement effective, scalable tech-enabled solutions to improve patient health."[170]

This is a shining example of how vertically partnering with a VC firm can serve a system's nonprofit mission and address a national challenge such as rural healthcare. First, Bassett leadership recognized that the solution to the challenges of rural healthcare requires a digital ecosystem. Second, Bassett likely did not have the up-front capital to fund this initiative or to hire the needed vendors. Third, Bassett likely did not have the internal technical, operational, and business expertise to deploy and maintain this initiative. But what the company did have was a really forward-thinking strategic vision to vertically partner with a VC firm.

Another shining example of the benefits of a VC-healthcare system partnership is Hartford HealthCare. In October 2022 Hartford

---

170 "Andreessen Horowitz Bio + Health Fund and Bassett Healthcare Network Leverage Digital Health to Address Rural Healthcare Needs," Business Wire, November 7, 2022, https://www.businesswire.com/news/home/20221107005388/en/.

HealthCare opened up its newly renovated 110,000-square-foot administrative headquarters, which resemble a Silicon Valley start-up. A few weeks later, it announced a partnership with two VC firms, Morningside Group and Connecticut Innovations. What's notable is that this wasn't their first such venture. In March 2020 they partnered with another venture fund, the Israel Innovation Authority. The reason for their thinking is plainly stated by CEO Dr. Jeffrey Flaks. "Embracing innovation is a central part of our culture and we needed to bring people together in an environment that could foster it."

Hartford's approach is to invite early-stage start-ups to work on pilot projects, for which the company sets clinical and financial goals. One example is start-up Wellink, whose product has significantly reduced readmissions in patients with chronic obstructive pulmonary disease. In addition to solving their clinical problems, Hartford has the opportunity to invest and partner with these start-ups, generating new revenue streams. Picking up on Dr. Flak's commentary, Dr. Barry Stein, Hartford's innovation officer, states it with simplicity, "We partner with start-ups to solve a problem in our organization.... If you're not investing in innovation, you're going to be behind and you're not going to survive."[171]

This approach is not limited to individual VC firms partnering with a single hospital system or provider group. For example, a VC firm that has emerged as a leader in working with healthcare systems is General Catalyst. In November 2022 General Catalyst announced that it had created a collaborative partnership with fifteen leading healthcare systems across the country, including academic medical centers and not-for-profit and for-profit hospital systems. Amazingly,

---

171 Gabriel Perna, "Health Systems Turn to Venture Capital amid Financial Challenges," *Modern Healthcare*, April 17, 2023, https://www.modernhealthcare.com/finance/health-systems-venture-capital-hartford-healthcare-general-catalyst.

these fifteen healthcare partners provide medical care to 10 percent of the American population across forty-three states.

General Catalyst's effort is unprecedented in its scope and boldness as they stated, "When we set out several years ago with the audaciously ambitious goal to transform the healthcare system, we knew we could never do it alone. No one company could 'disrupt' healthcare; it would require the creation of an ecosystem of partners, motivated behind a shared vision to create a system that was more accessible, proactive, and affordable. We didn't want to just catalyze change; we wanted to create a movement."[172]

General Catalyst has framed this collaborative venture as "personalized care at scale." It's a part of their larger "Health Assurance" movement, the stated objective of which is "creating a more proactive, affordable, and equitable system of care," with a specific agenda focused on the shift to aging in place and the home as the epicenter of care, reimagining the approach to rural health, transforming the healthcare workforce, operationalizing value-based care, empowering health equity, and accelerating innovations in the biologic medical sciences. One press release revealed the disruptive nature of this venture by describing the criteria for inclusion in this partnership: (1) a dissatisfaction with the way healthcare is currently being delivered, (2) a readiness to make significant shifts, (3) board engagement, and (4) a strategy based on triggering transformation. Those are telling criteria for 'beyond the walls' leadership.

---

172 Hemant Taneja, "Another Health Assurance Milestone: Announcing Our 15 Health System Partners," General Catalyst, November 15, 2022, https://www.generalcatalyst.com/perspectives/another-health-assurance-milestone-announcing-our-15-health-system-partners.

Multi-Hospital System Vertical Partnerships

Hospital-to-hospital collaborative ventures are a different type of vertical partnership. One remarkable example is a recently announced partnership between MetroHealth and the Medical University of South Carolina (MUSC). Together, they've formed a spin-off company, Ovatient, which aims to redesign the traditional care delivery model while maintaining connectivity to health systems' clinical expertise. Their focus is on developing virtual primary and specialty care as well as home-based care. The tagline for this new collaborative venture is an elegant counterpunch to the titans: "built by health systems, for health systems." It's a brilliant move to leverage their legacy standing and mission and to position themselves as a superior brand. They said,

> As nontraditional healthcare providers continue to enter the healthcare ecosystem, and seek to capitalize on digital technologies and the convenience they provide, MUSC Health & Metro Health are creating Ovatient to offer the same convenience and a better experience, all while preserving the connectivity to acute and procedural care sites so that patients do not endure fragmented care experiences.[173]

Here's a second example. In 2018 seven major health systems, including the Mayo Clinic and HCA, formed a 501(c)(4) social welfare organization, Civica Rx. Their goal was to make generic medications more readily available to hospital systems across the country. Drug shortages have been estimated to cost over half a billion dollars, and Civica Rx is directly mitigating those costs. Most recently, they've announced that three generic insulins will be available at much lower costs than other manufacturers. This move has caused large pharma-

---

173 "MUSC Health and the MetroHealth System Create Ovatient," MetroHealth, October 24, 2022, https://news.metrohealth.org/musc-health-and-the-metrohealth-system-create-ovatient/.

ceutical companies such as Eli Lilly to follow suit. Today one-third of all US hospital beds are partnered with Civica Rx.[174]

And here's one more example. Twenty-seven health systems, which cover 16 percent of all US healthcare spend, formed a clinical data company called Truveta. Together, they are normalizing and de-identifying their combined patient data, amassing the largest clinical data set available for research. Trinity Health CEO, Michael Slubowski, describes the value of this partnership: "We believe the cure for certain diseases could lie within the Truveta platform. For the first time in the history of health, we have enough data at scale to dramatically advance innovation in healthcare with collective commitment to partner on ethical innovation."[175]

Modeled after Civica Rx and Truveta, Graphite Health brought together a number of different health systems and philanthropies to create a digital health platform that allows for more rapid and secure development and adoption of digital health technologies. The current challenge is that healthcare systems are forced to build "point to point" integrations, which aren't scalable or affordable. For example, health systems spend, on average, two years implementing new digital tools. With Graphite Health, that timeline to adoption can be dramatically reduced because they are creating a marketplace that connects health systems (the buyers) with digital technology developers (the sellers) in a standard and secure infrastructure with "plug and play" interoperability. In addition, this multihealthcare system venture enables systems to rapidly test ideas before they commit significant resources to them. As Graphite Health CEO, Ries Robinson, put it, "As health systems, we have a once-in-a-lifetime opportunity to own our platform for the future. If we want to ensure that we prioritize our

---

174 Civica, accessed May 2, 2023, civicarx.org.

175 "Members," Truveta, https://www.truveta.com/members/.

patients and providers in every data-related process and transaction, we must seize it. The alternative: Ceding that authority to third parties with different motives."[176]

A Novel Multi-Hospital-Partnership Acquisition

A novel spin on multi-hospital vertical partnerships was announced in April 2023 by two highly integrated nonprofit health systems: Kaiser Permanente and Geisinger Health. While at the time of this writing the deal is still pending federal and state regulatory approvals, it is worth noting as another manifestation of the power of partnerships in the rapidly evolving "disrupted turned disruptor" landscape. On April 26, 2023, Kaiser Permanente (KP), announced its plan to acquire Geisinger Health (GH). At first glance, this acquisition seems to follow the well-worn pattern we previously discussed of hospital acquisitions and consolidations. KP is one of the largest healthcare systems in the country, with thirty-nine hospitals, nearly twenty-four thousand physicians, and 12.6 million insurance plan members in eight states and the District of Columbia, and a reported revenue of $95.4B last year.[177] GH is a ten-hospital system, employing more than 1,700 physicians with approximately 600,000 health plan members.[178]

But this is where the similarities end and the novelty begins. For starters, both organizations have had mature health plans in place for decades. In essence, they have been among the few hospital-based payviders in the country and are often held up as the industry gold

---

176 "An Introduction to Graphite Health," white paper, Graphite Health, accessed March 24, 2023, https://s3.amazonaws.com/external_clips/3379226/%282020-01-09%29_ Graphite_Health_White_Paper.pdf?1585675026.

177 Anna Wilde Mathews, "Health System Kaiser Permanente to Combine with Hospital Operator Geisinger," *Wall Street Journal*, April 26, 2023, https://www.wsj.com/articles/health-system-kaiser-permanente-to-combine-with-hospital-operator-geisinger-ee1c0edf.

178 Ibid.

standard for what integrated healthcare can look like. In addition to being payviders, both organizations have also been pioneering national leaders in the clinical quality movement, in addressing community-based social determinants of health, and in value-based care. The second differentiating attribute is that KP is not going to fold GH into itself or create a newly merged company. Instead, it is forming a separate entity named Risant Health. GH will be the first hospital system in this new nonprofit, and the plan is to add another four to six hospitals over the next five years. As Greg Adams, KP's CEO, states, "[It's] a way to really ensure that not-for-profit, value-based community health is not only alive but is thriving in this country."[179] It's a nontraditional merger in that Risant will operate independently and GH, along with the other hospital systems to join, will keep its name. Jaewon Ryu, GH's CEO is expected to be the chief executive at Risant once the deal goes through.

Now comes the third differentiating attribute. As more hospitals join Risant, it will serve to support them in their transition to and optimization of value-based care, essentially providing them with the decades of experience that both KP and GH have as value-based, integrated healthcare systems who own their own health plans. The stated goal is to target and acquire other hospitals and provider groups that are working toward the shift to value-based care. According to a GH press release, Risant Health's value-based platform will include "practices and capabilities in areas such as care model design, pharmacy, consumer digital engagement, health plan product development, and

---

179   Reed Abelson, "Kaiser Permanente to Acquire Geisinger," *New York Times*, April 26, 2023, https://www.nytimes.com/2023/04/26/health/kaiser-permanente-geisinger.html.

purchasing."[180] To support the effort, KP announced that it's planning to invest $5 billion in Risant over the next five years and expects to see revenues totaling $30 to $35 billion in that same time frame.[181]

It's important to underscore that this is a uniquely bold and future-facing approach to multi-hospital system partnerships. First, the merger is being structured as a separate and independent subsidiary of KP.[182] Some have suggested that this innovative and nontraditional iteration is a result of both KP's and GH's previous unsuccessful attempts at replication and expansion.[183] To be clear, far from viewing this as a criticism, I perceive this to be two leading organizations demonstrating resilience and adaptation—going beyond the walls.

Second, this new subsidiary is a nonprofit, multi-hospital endeavor dedicated to expanding and accelerating the shift to value-based care—promoting affordability, quality, and preventive care. While the deal serves the underlying financial and competitive growth needs of both organizations,[184] it is an unprecedented example of the power of partnership directed at the much-needed purpose of advancing value-based care in our country. It also represents a merger of titanic proportions as the larger consolidated entity will have over

---

180 "Kaiser Permanente and Geisinger Come Together to Launch Risant Health and Expand Access to Value-Based Care," Geisinger news releases, April 26, 2023, https://www.geisinger.org/about-geisinger/news-and-media/news-releases/2023/04/26/15/46/kaiser-permanente-and-geisinger-come-together-to-launch-risant-health.

181 Anna Wilde Mathews, "Health System Kaiser Permanente to Combine With Hospital Operator Geisinger," Wall Street Journal, April 26, 2023, https://www.wsj.com/articles/health-system-kaiser-permanente-to-combine-with-hospital-operator-geisinger-ee1c0edf.

182 Ibid.

183 Bob Herman, "New Mega-Deal Highlights Geisinger's Fall, and Raises Concerns about Where Kaiser Is Going Next," April 30, 2023, Stat News, https://www.statnews.com/2023/04/30/geisinger-kaiser-permanente-risant-strategy/?utm_campaign=health_care_inc&utm_medium=email&_hsmi=256420048&_hsenc=p2ANqtz-__AxKTQurhPEwpXtM8FGiVAhHk-RX2iDvvJ2a5UvT-w9li1-e6bCF8mwg_xKK_xdgzBM-NNNddUXGxsvG2ymArsBKTEQ&utm_content=256420048&utm_source=hs_email.

184 Ibid.

$100 billion in annual revenue, expanding KP's and GH's reach to more states and a broader patient population. Greg Adams, KP's CEO and chairman, captures the aim this way, "By helping other health systems achieve our value-based quality outcomes and savings in multi-payer, multi-provider environments, we believe Risant Health can deliver a transformative new solution to America's systemic health care problems. And, given its history in this space, we can think of no better organization than Geisinger to be the inaugural health system to join Risant Health."[185]

DIRECT-TO-EMPLOYER HOSPITAL-BASED PARTNERSHIPS

In chapter 7 we did a deep dive into the Transcarent platform. We spent quite a bit of time focused on the employer-as-customer side of things. But we didn't really touch on the other side of that platform, the supplier side, which, in this case, is largely based on hospital systems.

To set the stage here, let's do a quick historical overview of the direct-to-employer (DTE) movement.

For years, there have been employer coalitions such as the Pacific Business Group on Health and the National Business Group on Health. These organizations, similar to the Walmart employer example, have essentially measured the variation in care outcomes and costs and directed contracts to healthcare systems and providers of higher value. Although these endeavors generated tremendous

---

185 "Kaiser Permanente and Geisinger Come Together to Launch Risant Health and Expand Access to Value-Based Care," Geisinger News Releases, April 26, 2023, https://www.geisinger.org/about-geisinger/news-and-media/news-releases/2023/04/26/15/46/kaiser-permanente-and-geisinger-come-together-to-launch-risant-health.

data and understanding, it's unclear that they had a measurable or sustained impact either on the outsize rise in healthcare costs for employers or on marked improvements in outcomes.[186] These much-needed employer-led coalitions were ahead of their time, but they were also lacking a cohesive platform.

In addition to the employer-led coalitions, there have also existed DTE contractual relationships between individual hospital systems and local employers. Hospital-based healthcare systems have, for years, been contracting directly with small local employers, midsize regional employers, and even large national employers. The Willis Towers Watson 23rd Annual Best Practices in Health Care Employer Survey found that 22 percent of employers (with at least one thousand employees) were using or highly considering direct contracting.[187]

While these direct contracting relationships have been satisfactory at the local level, they cannot accommodate the needs of corporations with a national footprint. National employers would need to negotiate, maintain, and monitor multiple contracts with multiple hospital systems across the country—a formidable task for both the national employers and the regional healthcare systems. In response to this unmet market need, there have been attempts over the past few years to construct nationwide hospital coalitions to service national employers with footprints in multiple regions and cities across the country. To date, these efforts have been unsuccessful.

Enter Transcarent into this rapidly evolving scenario. As we discussed in chapter 7, Transcarent has constructed a technologically sophisticated and consumer-oriented business platform. On the supplier side of their platform, Transcarent is curating and partnering

---

186 Zeev Neuwirth, *Reframing Healthcare: A Roadmap For Creating Disruptive Change* (Charleston: Advantage Media Group, 2019).

187 "Willis Towers Watson 23rd Annual Best Practices in Health Care Employer Survey," 2018, https://www.harmonyhealth.com/wp-content/uploads/2021/04/willis-towers-watson-23rd-annual-best-practices-in-health-care-employer-survey-full-report.pdf.

with high-quality healthcare systems and provider groups across the country. They've recently begun to refer to their approach as "Ecosystems of Excellence." Glen captures the value proposition for this new DTE ecosystem approach as follows: "Too often, the major obstacle ... is friction from third party middlemen and a lack of unbiased information, trusted guidance and easy access to care.... Transcarent offers employers ... the opportunity to provide a simpler, more satisfying experience for their employees by giving them the information and guidance to make the right care choices for their needs."[188]

The value proposition to employers and their employees is apparent. From the hospital (supplier) side, the opportunity and value proposition in this DTE ecosystem partnership is considerable and multifold. First, it represents an additional channel for hospitals to acquire new patients from a large regional and national employer base, including patients who are in need of higher-volume, higher-margin services such as in orthopedics, cardiology, bariatrics, oncology, and women's health. Second, it diversifies hospitals' revenue streams away from the traditional payer contracts, which could also provide additional negotiating leverage. Third, it promises to greatly reduce the significant administrative hassles and costly payment delays that have long plagued hospital systems and provider groups in their relationship with insurance carrier payers. Finally, it will more easily allow for payment to healthcare systems for services that fall outside of the traditional payer contracts—services such as virtual and digital health, home-based care, navigation and coordination services, and lifestyle medicine programs such as weight management. The DTE ecosystem approach clearly represents a mutually beneficial opportu-

---

188 "Rush University System for Health Selects Transcarent to Provide New Digital Health and Care Experience to Enhance Medical Plan Benefits," Business Wire, February 18, 2022, https://www.businesswire.com/news/home/20220218005031/en/Rush-University-System-for-Health-Selects-Transcarent-to-Provide-New-Digital-Health-and-Care-Experience-to-Enhance-Medical-Plan-Benefits.

nity for hospital systems, for employers, and for their employees and dependents. It also represents a potential threat to the payviders who are aggressively competing in the commercial employer market.

There are numerous companies out there that are disruptors in the DTE market. It's an entire industry segment. For example, Carrum Health is building a national network of Centers of Excellence where they have negotiated a bundled, set price for surgical procedures as well as some cancer care. They then sell those bundles directly to employers and provide wraparound patient support services, including an initial clinical consultation with top-tier physicians. And Quantum Health provides health navigators for employees to best use their employer-provided health benefits.

The take-home point here is that the DTE market represents significant partnership opportunities, as well as meaningful revenue diversification and margin enhancement, for hospital-based health-care systems.

Let's now explore another type of vertical partnership that also goes beyond the walls in a big way. This one occurs between a leading healthcare system and a national retailer.

A HOSPITAL-RETAILER VERTICAL PARTNERSHIP

In March 2023 Best Buy and Atrium Health officially announced a partnership. The story was highlighted by national news media outlets, including CNBC, *Good Morning America*, *Forbes*, and *Fortune* largely because it signaled that Best Buy was expanding into healthcare. The morning show hosts joked about picking up a wide-screen TV and a heart monitor at the same time. Cute, but they missed the punchline. The real story here was that for the first time, a partnership had been forged between a national retailer (Best Buy) and a large healthcare system (Atrium Health, now part of Advocate Health, the fifth largest healthcare system in the country). A partnership to codevelop the home-based care ecosystem.

Both organizations had already spent years developing their own internal strategies around virtual care, digital care, and home-based care prior to the partnership discussions. Atrium Health, with nearly a decade of experience in virtual care, had launched virtual visits, e-visits, and automated visits, as well as virtual specialty consults to dozens of its hospitals, particularly its rural hospitals. Atrium Health also had a mature and robust home care program with a fleet of paramedics, mobile units, home nursing programs, skilled nursing facilities, and durable medical equipment services.

In 2018 Best Buy, under the leadership of CEO Corie Barry, made a strategic decision to launch a healthcare division (Best Buy Health) and acquired well over a billion dollars' worth of healthcare assets. These included a phenomenal national caring center, GreatCall, and their line of personal assist devices for seniors, as well as Critical Signal Technologies' Personal Emergency Response Systems (PERS) assist devices and their specialized services addressing seniors' SDOH. In 2021 Best Buy also acquired Current Health, one of the premier remote patient monitoring service companies.

In coming together, their mission was to codevelop a home-based care ecosystem that would not only serve Atrium's patient population but could also be adapted to serve other healthcare systems. The stated goal was to enable providers in delivering high-quality care to patients in the comfort of their own homes while helping to reduce the emotional and financial burdens on patients and caregivers.[189]

---

189 Bruce Jaspen, "Best Buy Pushes Deeper into Healthcare with 'Hospital at Home' Partnership," *Forbes*, March 7, 2023, https://www.forbes.com/sites/bruce-japsen/2023/03/07/best-buy-pushes-deeper-into-healthcare-with-home-care-partnership/?sh=59e504412c83.

There are a number of characteristics that make this a novel vertical partnership. First, this is a complementary partnership, not a client-vendor relationship. What Best Buy brings to the partnership includes their omnichannel retail footprint and retail capabilities, their premier remote monitoring devices and reporting platform, a world-class supply chain and logistics platform, and their Geek Squad service adapted to support patient education and to enable health technologies in the home. What Atrium Health brings to the partnership includes their nationally renowned clinical expertise; a pioneering, enterprise-wide virtual care program; an established and nationally leading hospital at home program; and multiple postacute care services.

Second, there is cultural alignment between both organizations, including their deep commitments to addressing healthcare disparities and inequities. This cultural alignment was expressed publicly by Deborah DiSanzo, Best Buy Health's president, in the following statement: "We knew Atrium Health was the right partner to help tackle the unique challenges within the care at home experience.... The holistic combination of resources ... will change the lives of consumers and enable them to heal right in their own homes, surrounded by the people and things they love the most ... enabl[ing] care in the home for everyone."[190] And as Dr. Rasu Shrestha, chief innovation and commercialization officer at Atrium Health, added, "This is the coming together of technology and empathy."[191]

Third, this partnership addresses all three domains of 'beyond the walls'—extending care beyond the literal walls of the hospital and

---

190   Jaspen, "Best Buy Pushes Deeper into Healthcare with 'Hospital at Home' Partnership."

191   "Atrium Health and Best Buy Health Partner to Enhance Hospital at Home Experience," Atrium Health News, March 2023, https://atriumhealth.org/dailydose/2023/03/06/atrium-health-and-best-buy-health-partner-to-enhance-hospital-at-home-experience.

clinic, transcending the conceptual walls by focusing on the whole health of patients and families in the context of their homes, and engaging the systemic level by leveraging digital platforms and vertical partnering.

A *PLATFORM* FOR VERTICAL PARTNERSHIPS

Imagine if multiple innovative organizations could be based in one 'beyond the walls' hub. Well, they can, and it's called an Innovation District. These districts exist in a few cities across the country, including Boston, Houston, and Philadelphia. These hubs are built within a real estate development in which multiple corporate colocated tenants from industry, research, education, and government come together to create a hotbed of scientific advancement and economic development. It's the rich diversity and complementarity that creates the potential for cross-fertilizations and collaborations, leading to new research, new discoveries, new business ventures, and new products and services. One of the newest and most innovative of these districts is called "the Pearl." Based in Charlotte, North Carolina, the Pearl broke ground in early 2023 as a cutting-edge initiative launched by Atrium Health (now a part of Advocate Health) and Wexford Science & Technology. There are a number of unique aspects of this particular innovation district worth noting.

1. The Pearl's initial (anchor) tenant, IRCAD, is a preeminent research and education institute specializing in computer-assisted, robotic, laparoscopic surgical procedures. IRCAD has been described as a mecca for surgeons and will act as a "super magnet" for attracting corporate entities, surgeons, and entrepreneurs from across the country as well as inter-

nationally.[192] Charlotte will be the exclusive North American site for IRCAD, adding to its attractiveness.

2. The Pearl innovation district will be connected to an existing "innovation quarter" (IQ) based in Winston-Salem, located less than eighty miles north of Charlotte. The IQ was cocreated with Wake Forest Baptist Health, now a part of Atrium Health. In addition to collaborating with the IQ, IRCAD and the other entities in the Pearl can expand their collaboration with Wake Forest Baptist Health's other clinical, research, and commercialization capabilities. This regional collaborative will form a novel "innovation corridor."

3. The Pearl innovation district has a profound academic base. It will be the home to the Charlotte campus of the Wake Forest Medical School (Charlotte's first four-year medical school) and will also collaborate with the Wake Forest School of Professional Studies and its Business School, as well as the Carolinas College of Health Sciences.

4. The Pearl is explicitly focused on diversity, equity, and inclusion. In fact, the name, *the Pearl,* was selected to honor the thriving Black American "Brooklyn" community that existed in Charlotte's Second Ward for years. That community was razed in the 1960s and 1970s as part of an "urban renewal" project. One can't change history, but the commitment of the Pearl is to change the future, and one way of doing that is by not forgetting the heritage of the past. Gene Woods, CEO of Advocate Health, captures this commitment well. "Many might say this area of town and its

---

192 Elise Franco and Lillian Johnson, "Atrium Breaks Ground on New Wake Forest Med School and Innovation District in Midtown Charlotte," *Triad Business Journal,* January 18, 2023.

rich history have been largely overlooked. But we're here now to begin a new chapter to this story and honor this special place as we empower the neighborhoods around it, which are shaped by diverse people and perspectives, rooted in inclusivity and belonging, and filled with endless potential."[193]

5. The twenty-acre Pearl district will include spaces available to the entire community, as well as affordable housing developments, in an effort to transform the future through the economic development and support of local communities. It's expected that this district will add 12,000 jobs to the greater Charlotte region, and 5,500 of those will be within the innovation district itself. It's expected that 30 to 40 percent of those jobs will not require a college degree.

I've described the Pearl as an innovation district, an economic development, an innovation corridor, a super magnet, and a national as well as international healthcare epicenter. But these attributes still don't fully depict what it actually is. The Pearl is a multifaceted *platform* that will attract vendors and customers for the sharing, incubation, and commercialization of ideas, products, and services. As you'll recall from chapter 7, one of the characteristics of platforms is their network effect. As more companies and individuals join, the platform's value proposition increases. What distinguishes the Pearl from the other examples in this chapter is that it's much more than a vertical partnership. It's an entrepreneurial community

> As more companies and individuals join, the platform's value proposition increases.

---

193 "Introducing Charlotte's Innovation District: 'The Pearl,'" Atrium Health, March 3, 2023, https://atriumhealth.org/about-us/newsroom/news/2022/03/introducing-charlottes-innovation-district-the-pearl.

platform that will scale small businesses and generate novel combinations of partnerships and ventures. It is truly a 'beyond the walls' phenomena.

The examples in this chapter—all emerging from within legacy hospital-based healthcare systems—mark the beginning of a new 'beyond the walls' era in American healthcare. They're a fitting end to this chapter and this book. My hope is that all of the examples inspire and catalyze more innovations, partnerships, and platforms that empower us to greatly advance healthcare in America.

A STARTER TAXONOMY FOR HOSPITAL SYSTEM PARTNERSHIPS

- Vertical Partnerships
- Venture Capital Partnerships
- Multi-hospital system vertical partnerships
- A novel multi-hospital-partnership acquisition
- Direct-to-Employer hospital-based partnerships
- A hospital-retailer vertical partnership
- A platform for vertical partnerships

EPILOGUE
A CALL TO ACTION

*If you want something new, you have
to stop doing something old.*
–Peter Drucker

MY PURPOSE IN WRITING this book was to shed light and
a discerning perspective on the emerging realities of our healthcare
system. It's a positive outlook—all based in reality and not on con-
jecture or unfounded predictions. I'm hopeful about the future of
American healthcare, but I would label my perspective as "cautiously
optimistic."

It's important to recognize that the developments we've discussed
are already changing our direct experience and the outcomes of
healthcare. I don't know exactly what American healthcare will look
like five to seven years from now, but I firmly believe it's going to be
shockingly different than today. As I stated in chapter 1, I believe
we're going to see healthcare become much more decentralized, disag-
gregated, and democratized, leading to care that is more contextualized, customized, and connected. By 2030 American healthcare will
likely resemble what I've described in this book, and it will be much
more congruent with other facets of our life. By that I mean it will be

some sort of mashup of how we engage with and experience our cell phones, social media, streaming entertainment, and online retail and travel—more convenient, more accessible, more transparent, more consumer oriented, and more affordable. But again, given the walls that have been built up over the past century, it won't happen without intentional action and without us getting beyond the walls.

In a book like this, with so many examples of change, I felt it important to offer a few take-home points:

1. We will not advance healthcare and health in our country if we don't redesign, reorganize, and resource it differently.

   We need to get beyond the limits of the past and reframe healthcare with new orientations. We need to do more of what was highlighted in this book, building on the positive disruptive momentum that already exists. In the Supplement, I outline what this reframe road map looks like. Far from being a theoretical construct, the road map distills the path that I've observed dozens of 'beyond the walls' entrepreneurial leaders using.

2. If we want a healthcare system that works for us, that takes care of us, *all* of us, it will require us to overcome the inertia of the past.

   Leadership in healthcare, and in our country, needs to stop promoting and defending legacy approaches and begin removing the obstacles standing in the way of advancement. I began this book with a story about a successful 'beyond the walls' healthcare entrepreneur, Sean Duffy. Sean reviewed parts of the book as it was going through the final edit, and here's what he wrote back:

What dawns on me is that the "outside the walls" risk is even more harrowing in healthcare than in other industries: regulations, slow sales cycles, huge capital requirements, and extreme inertia against change. The net effect is that you have to be even crazier to step outside the walls in healthcare. The risk of "death" is significantly higher than in other entrepreneurial areas, which are already extremely high. Also, the healthcare community is far less likely to welcome you back.

3. Incumbent stakeholders and their leadership need to actively participate in creating change. If you're not part of the 'beyond the walls' solution, you're part of the 'behind the walls' problem.

    Change like this is disruptive and hard. We all have seemingly more immediate issues on our plates. There is an inevitable short-term loss for the stakeholders, but there is no gain without pain, and there is no creation without some destruction. One of the hallmarks of a tipping point is when the pain of the present becomes greater than the pain of change. I believe we're rapidly approaching that tipping point, if not already upon it.

The reality of our current situation is this: there is no fairy tale ending. It's going to take hard work to tip the scales, and it's going to require a great deal of energy and integrity to make the transition to a new era in healthcare delivery. More to the point, it's going to take real leadership—leadership that stands up, speaks out, and demands a better and more affordable healthcare system.

MOVING BEYOND "IT'S NEVER THE RIGHT TIME" TO "THE TIME IS NOW"

A few months ago, I gave a talk—and one of the executive physician leaders in attendance raised his hand to ask a question.

"Dr. Neuwirth, with all due respect, how do you expect us to invest in these disruptive changes when times are so hard? Hospitals, healthcare systems, and practices are facing unprecedented revenue pressures, cost pressures, and staffing pressures. We're all burned out. *Now* cannot be the right time to make the changes you're talking about!"

"Well," I responded, "I hear you and don't want to make light of any of the serious problems you were just mentioning. And if I were new to healthcare, I might be swayed by your argument. But I'm not new to healthcare. The problem with your argument is this: Three or four years ago, prepandemic, I heard a smart, successful, and practical leader just like you say something along the lines of 'Zeev, how do you expect us to invest in these changes when times are so *good?* Hospitals, healthcare systems, and practices are facing incredible revenues and profits. *Why would we change now?* So the problem with your argument, and his argument, and every similar argument I've heard over the past three decades boils down to this: *according to you all, it's never a good time to change our healthcare system.*"

And here's the red herring. The issue is not a financial one, as these arguments seem to suggest. It's actually a leadership issue. As leaders, all of us have a choice to make. We can make choices based on our current circumstances, largely using them as excuses. Or we can make choices based on our principles and commitments. We can make choices based on short-term gain, maintaining the current system for as long as we can. Or we can make choices based on our stated purpose and pledge to advance the health and well-being of our patients and communities to the best of our abilities.

What we need, what our patients need, what the American public needs are healthcare leaders who are choosing to make decisions from their commitment. I'm not saying it's easy. In fact, it's anything but easy. But it's necessary if we are going to get beyond the walls. Without this kind of visionary leadership, we are going to be in deep trouble in the long run. And I think we are seeing some of that play itself out right now.

For far too long, we have kicked the can down the road when it comes to making significant changes to our healthcare system, perhaps waiting for the "right" time, which will never come or perhaps waiting for some definitive proof, which will also never come. Recently, I sat in on a webinar, "The Role of Business in Improving Health and Health Equity: A Workshop," sponsored by the National Academy of Science, Engineering, and Medicine. My colleague, Terry Williams, was facilitating it and had invited me to listen in. There was one discussion in particular that I found gripping. Dr. Greg Fairchild, a professor at the University of Virginia School of Business and dean and CEO of UVA Northern Virginia, was one of the panelists. Despite having a strong academic background, there is nothing academic about Dr. Fairchild's views. He's been working at the intersection of business management and healthcare for years, and he has a grounded and practical take on things.

What I immediately admired about him was that he didn't mince words. He said there wasn't enough thorough research on the effectiveness of many of the healthcare breakthroughs—new business, payment, and care delivery models—to take an academically sound position. He went on to say "We're at the edge. We're in the present moment. We're ahead of any scientific or rigorous study of any of these things we're talking about or most of the things we're talking about. The best we can do is look at the exemplars, look at the examples of what is already happening that is working and that is bringing us in a positive direction."

The word "exemplar" resonated with me, and his statement gripped me: "The best we can do is look at the exemplars, look at the examples of what is already happening that is working and that is bringing us in a positive direction." I could not have articulated a better description of what I had been doing for the past several years of my career. This has been the goal of my in-depth interviews and is the purpose of this book. I have been identifying and studying these 'beyond the walls' exemplars in our healthcare system with the explicit goal of sharing their positive deviance, spreading the word in the hope that it will catalyze more creative dialogue and game-changing action. In these pages you have heard directly from outstanding exemplars who are creating change and showing us a way forward. You have learned for yourself about their personal and professional journeys and their commitment to advancing American healthcare delivery. My hope is that they inform and inspire us all to do more of the same—to get beyond the walls.

THE COURAGE TO BEGIN AGAIN

This journey of discovering the exemplars and the 'beyond the walls' leaders has enlightened and energized me. It has emboldened me to speak out and to act out. My intention in writing this second book was to share that journey with you in the hope that it incites you to channel your creative energies into productive humanistic transformative change. If you are reading these words, I'll wager that you're already a transformative leader—an exemplar—or on the way to becoming one.

I recently came across the theory that the only thing that can disrupt a pattern is another pattern. The type of leadership I've been studying is leadership that lays down new patterns—leadership that advances beyond the walls literally, conceptually, and systemically. And we are beginning to see how effective that leadership can be. The old patterns in healthcare are being disrupted by new patterns. But our job is not yet done.

We have come to the end of this book, but we are just at the beginning of a new era in healthcare. Elie Wiesel, author, scholar, and Nobel Peace Prize Laureate, wrote, "When God created us, God gave Adam and Eve a secret—and that secret was not how to begin, but how to begin again." Well, we can begin again with our healthcare system. But we must keep in mind that "beginning again" is not about merely improving on what existed before. It is about divergent reframes that tap into our deeply human ability to let go of the past, to transform the present, and to begin a new future.

To begin anew will require courage. I've been observing, appreciating, and experiencing the courage it takes to do this work. One way you could understand this book is as a collection of stories about courage. My working definition of courage is that it's a tipping point, a shift in an equation when an individual's or group's sense of purpose becomes greater than their fear of the consequences. The entrepreneurs and leaders, the exemplars in this book, exhibit that tipping point. It's a visceral subtext that runs throughout the stories I've shared.

One of the most enlightening comments I've heard about courage came from a recent interview I conducted with Dr. Don Berwick, who is one of the most courageous and impactful healthcare luminaries of our time. He shared this quote from C. S. Lewis: "Courage is not simply one of the virtues but the form of every virtue at the testing point." I believe we are all being tested, at every point along the way, as we attempt to transcend our current situation, as we attempt to get beyond the walls of our current healthcare system. It takes visionary leadership to *see* beyond the walls, but it takes courageous leadership to *travel* beyond them. My hope is that this book has provided you with examples and exemplars that inspire you to bring all of your virtues together, to allow yourself to be tested, to release your courageous spirit, and to attain the purpose you've set out for yourself. Go beyond the walls, my friends, and lead us toward all that you discover.

> It takes visionary leadership to *see* beyond the walls, but it takes courageous leadership to *travel* beyond them.

AN UPDATE ON REFRAMING HEALTHCARE[194]

*Whatever situation we are in, by reframing it
we can change our entire response, giving us
the strength to survive, the courage to persist,
and the resilience to emerge, on the far side of
darkness, into the light of a new and better day.*

–Rabbi Lord Jonathan Sacks

I BEGAN CONDUCTING in-depth interviews with healthcare entrepreneurs and leaders in 2016. At the time I wanted to understand not only what they were doing but also *how* they were doing it—their mindsets, their approaches, their strategies, and their tactics—so as to guide myself and others in how to transcend the limiting walls of our healthcare system.

After meticulously studying forty or fifty of these interviews, I began to recognize commonalities. During one interview, I found myself a bit exasperated and literally blurted out to my guest, "What is it with you all? It's like someone handed you the same exact playbook,

---

194 Neuwirth, *Reframing Healthcare.*

one that I didn't get!" Needless to say, he was a bit surprised at the non sequitur and asked me what I was talking about. I collected myself and responded, "It's like you're all following the same handbook."

At that point I had yet to grasp the concept of reframing or discern the steps. But I could distinguish a common pathway, a basic protocol that was different from any that I had studied, trained in, or even had familiarity with. It took me another couple of years of analyzing dozens and dozens more of these interviews to recognize that they were all utilizing a process I ended up calling "reframing." I began to decipher the steps of this protocol and then to test my theory with each successive leader that I interviewed.

What emerged from this study were three defining characteristics that differentiate reframing from other approaches. First, it requires us to **reorient** our thinking toward a different way of making sense of the world. Second, it requires us to understand the problem from that new orientation and therefore **redefine** the problem. This is the hallmark of reframing. If you can't redefine the problem clearly, you haven't reframed it. And third, it requires us to **redirect** our strategies, tactics, and resources—to act within that new orientation and to pursue solutions that address the redefined problem.

Reframing is not a new concept. It has deep roots in the traditions of philosophy, religion, science, military strategy, and business.[195] Apparently, the Buddhists have been practicing the art of reframing for over two millennia. I learned that in a 2021 documentary titled *Mission Joy: Finding Happiness in Troubled Times*, in which the Dalai Lama explains reframing to Archbishop Desmond Tutu. During one of their recorded dialogues, the archbishop, listening to the Dalai Lama's story of the exodus from his homeland, remarked that it must have been very painful to become a permanent refugee from Tibet.

---

195   Neuwirth, *Reframing Healthcare*, chapter 2.

The Dalai responds with a wide smile and a surprising response: "So I personally prefer the refugee life. It's more useful. More opportunity to learn. More experience … if you look from one angle, you think how bad, how sad. But if you look from another angle … about that same event … ah, that gives me some new opportunity."

At that point in the documentary, they flash to Thupten Jinpa Langri, the Dalai's translator—a former Tibetan monk and an academic in religious studies—who goes on to explain "You see, cognitive reframing is a powerful technique to change your mindset, and in the Buddhist language we call it 'outlook.' This is a fundamental insight in Buddhist psychology. That's why so much emphasis is placed in Buddhist philosophy on changing the way you see the world … reframing can help us, liberate us." I had personally never heard of reframing before I discovered it in the interviews I conducted. To learn that it was a 2,500-year-old Buddhist practice further strengthened my conviction that reframing was a powerful process for transformation.

The Stoic philosophers have also been practicing the art of reframing since the writings of Marcus Aurelius in the first century. The fundamental reframe in stoicism is to see life's problems and challenges as opportunities for learning and growth—not to be avoided but appreciated, embraced, and addressed. The thirteenth-century Sufi poet Rumi deeply understood the art of reframing, as exemplified in so many of his writings. For example, in his poem "The Guest House," he reframes what are typically considered negative emotions and experiences such as depression, dark thoughts, shame, malice, and sorrow. Instead, he describes them as "guides from beyond," as welcomed and honorable guests that "may be clearing you out for some new delight." Rumi's poetry evokes a visceral appreciation of what a reframe feels like—a gut feeling I've experienced in most of the podcast interviews I've conducted over the past seven years.

When someone is actually reframing, it isn't just a cerebral act; it's an emotional and spiritual one as well.

At the core of cognitive behavioral therapy (CBT) is also this notion of reframing. In fact, for those who have studied the subject or are familiar with CBT, you might be experiencing an "aha moment" right now. CBT is all about taking the ways we think and creating a new orientation and, out of that orientation, new emotions and new behaviors. It can be applied to everything from changing your diet to smoking cessation, to addressing and overcoming phobias, to enhancing your relationships. CBT utilizes reframing as a tool to help us relieve our suffering by shifting our thoughts and therefore changing our very physiology. Again, reframing is not just in the head; it's a visceral activity when it's actually accomplished.

A historical reference for reframing in the realm of science is what has come to be known as a "paradigm shift." This term was made famous in a 1961 book by Thomas Kuhn titled *The Structure of Scientific Revolutions*.[196] In this landmark text, he brilliantly outlines the process of scientific revolutions in myriad scientific fields. What he describes as a paradigm shift is, in essence, the process of reframing.

Fundamentally, the process of reframing requires us to understand our situation from a different perspective in order to shake ourselves free from the implicit rules and biases of our current thinking and outlook. You can't always change your current reality, but you *can* change how you *perceive* and *respond* to that reality. It's that reframing that leads to the deployment of new solutions and the creation of a new reality.

I discovered all of this not by studying the Stoics or Buddhism or psychology or the history of science. I uncovered it by listening

---

196 Thomas Kuhn, *The Structure of Scientific Revolutions* (Chicago: University of Chicago Press, 1996).

intently and openly to hundreds of successful entrepreneurs, founders, and C-suite leaders, by listening to 'beyond the walls' thinkers and doers. So let me introduce you to the reframe roadmap, a tool for transformation that's been used by world-class leaders, scientists, philosophers, artists, and entrepreneurial trailblazers for two millennia—a transformation playbook that has certainly withstood the test of time and a playbook that is being used to transform American healthcare.

THE REFRAME ROAD MAP

In the first three years of interviewing, I discerned seven steps in what I called the "Reframe Road Map." For a more detailed explanation, please refer back to *Reframing Healthcare*. Here are those initial seven steps: (1) **reorient** our thinking, (2) **redefine** our problems, (3) **rebrand** our value proposition, (4) **redesign** our products and services, (5) establish our new set of **results** and performance metrics, (6) **reorganize** our current structures, and (7) **redirect our** strategies, tactics, and resources.

Since the publication of that book over four years ago, I've utilized the reframe road map more and subsequently simplified the approach into a three-act play: act 1—reorient and redefine, act 2—redesign, and act 3—reorganize and resource.

Act 1 contains two steps: **reorient** and **redefine**. These steps are conceptual in nature and begin with reorienting ourselves to a situation we're already familiar with. This requires creating a new narrative by taking a fresh and truer perspective on the subject at hand, one that is free of old, outworn assumptions and prejudices and, at the same time, adds to the mix new knowledge and expertise from different fields.

Often, when people try to change a system from within, they're blocked by a conceptual brick wall that has writ large on it: "But this is the way we've always done things." A naive outsider, on the other hand, can walk into a dysfunctional operation, immediately recognize its dysfunction, and wonder why no one has attempted to correct it. This is exactly what reorienting is all about, which is why it often does require an outsider or someone from a different discipline or industry to provide a new take on things.

After we reorient, we are now able to redefine the problems at hand. And this is one of the differentiations between reimagining or rethinking and reframing. If you can't redefine the problem, then you have not reframed it. It's almost a litmus test. You have to be able to say "Hmmm, I see the problem differently" and articulate what that new problem definition is. We spend most of our time and energy trying to solve the same problems in the same ways instead of finding a different way of looking at those problems. The *Harvard Business Review* uses the example of the manager of an apartment building getting constant complaints about a slow elevator. The solution that would occur to most of us is make the elevator faster—put in a new motor, whatever it takes. The solution that probably would not occur to us is to make the elevator ride *feel* shorter. For example, by putting mirrors on the walls of the elevator car, people will be distracted by looking at themselves and will actually complain less.[197] What's really interesting about the mirror solution is it doesn't actually solve the problem in the way it was originally framed, as the article puts it: "It doesn't make the elevator faster. Instead, it proposes a different understanding of the problem." In other words, the problem was reframed and *redefined*, which made a simpler alternative solution possible.

---

197   Thomas Wedell-Wedellsborg, "Are You Solving the Right Problems?" *Harvard Business Review*, January–February 2017, https://hbr.org/2017/01/are-you-solving-the-right-problems.

Act 1 is necessary and critical for the reframing of healthcare, but it is not sufficient. If you only get as far as Act 1, you get stuck in the "this is a new day" phenomena—a lot of hope and hoopla but no follow-through. This is something I've observed numerous times throughout my career. There's a reorientation and even a redefining, but not much substance follows that. This is why the notion of reimagining healthcare is an incomplete one. It can also be demoralizing. How many times have you heard that phrase "reimagining healthcare"? I'll be honest with you. I ran a campaign in 2006–2007 called "reimagine healthcare." I only wish I had been aware of all of the steps of the reframe road map that are required to make that reimagining a reality.

Act 2 of the reframe road map involves **redesign**. Design is an established discipline that impacts almost every facet of our lives as consumers. Think about each product you come into contact with every day: the morning alarm, the toothbrush, the showerhead, the shampoo bottle, your kitchen appliances, your car, the device in your hand. All of those things have been expertly designed. Even the food we eat has been designed by chefs, food scientists, and professional designers who are experts in taste, smell, and texture. A successful redesign has a huge impact on a consumer. And the hallmarks of successful design include desirability, feasibility, and viability. Good designs must be aesthetically appealing. They must meet functional and emotional and relational needs. They must be simple, preferably convenient, and user-friendly. They must be feasible in that they must work, given the available technologies, operational, and business models. And they must be viable on a financial level.

While Act 2 is necessary, it, too, is insufficient if that's all you do. Redesigning healthcare without Act 1 or 3 often ends up in largely cosmetic changes. For example, a company may change its logo without changing how it does business and decide that's all it needs to do, even though nothing essential has changed. You can redesign the traditional hospital, and that would be a really nice and important thing to do, but reframing the hospital would be transformational. And if you stop at Act 2, you will end up with "pilot-itis." I've heard it said, jokingly, that there are more pilots in healthcare than there are in the airline industry. Many of us in healthcare have wondered why so many pilots in healthcare don't get scaled and are unsustainable. Now some don't deserve to get deployed, and that is the purpose of a pilot or prototype phase. But many, if not most, pilots don't make it out of that stage because they stop at Act 2 of the reframe road map.

Act 3 is invaluable but often misunderstood—organizations stop before this stage and never take the required actions that will create replicable, scalable, and sustainable progress. The first scene of Act 3 is **reorganizing**. If you've reoriented your thinking, redefined the problem, and redesigned the solution, it will almost certainly require that you reorganize your operations to maintain and sustain the new approach. It's all about people, process, policies, and technology. We might have to reorganize our divisions or our processes. We might need to put new policies and protocols in place. And technology, as we've seen throughout this book, is the great enabler of reframing.

The second scene of Act 3 is **resourcing**. I often liken this phase to having a rocket ship on the launchpad but forgetting to fuel it. This is the commitment phase. It's the reorganizing of how we spend our valuable assets and resources. To put it bluntly, it's all about putting our money where our mouths are. If you want to really know what an organization is about, look at how they spend their money and look at how they bonus their executives. That's Act 3. If you don't do Acts 1 and 2 and instead simply reorganize, what I call that is "reorganizing the chairs on the deck of the titanic." You look like you're busy, and you look like you're going somewhere, but you're not going anywhere good.

I've shared this reframe road map with dozens of organizations over the past five years. I usually get nodding heads, and their leaders will admit that when they've attempted to initiate meaningful transformative change, they've skipped steps and even whole stages of the reframing process to the detriment of their organization's progress. On the other hand, the successful entrepreneurs and leaders I've been interviewing over the past seven years not only nod their head in agreement; they can also point out exactly how they've gone through each of these stages.

The Future of Healthcare Is Here and Now

There are three final thoughts I'd like to share with you in this *Reframing Healthcare* update.

First, there's that famous quote by science fiction writer William Gibson: "The future is already here. It's just not evenly distributed yet." One thing to recognize about every single innovation described in this book is that they are not about what *might* happen. They describe what is already happening. It's up to us to figure out how to spread them more broadly and more equitably.

Second, I hope you've recognized the steps of reframing in the 'beyond the walls' examples I've curated in this book. But more than that, I hope you recognize how you are already a part of the 'beyond the walls' movement, whether as a provider, patient, payer, policy maker, administrator, or any other stakeholder impacted by or impacting American healthcare.

Third, the act of reframing is especially suited for solving problems that are seemingly unsolvable and for addressing situations in which the way we've been doing things doesn't seem to extricate us from the dilemma we've been stuck in. The renowned business leader and HBS professor Clayton Christensen captured this brilliantly when he wrote, "When the business world encounters an intractable management problem, it's a sign that ... there isn't yet a satisfactory theory for what's causing the problem, and under what circumstances it can be overcome."[198]

It's obvious that we are precisely in that sort of situation in American healthcare and have been for decades. If the problem were easily fixed within our current framework, it likely would have been solved by now, given all of the resources and expertise that have been brought to bear. More to the point, if we could solve it through our current paradigms and approaches, we already would have.

---

198 Clayton Christensen, *The Innovator's Dilemma: When New Technologies Cause Great Firms to Fail* (Boston: Harvard Business School Press, 1997).

ACKNOWLEDGMENTS

I COULD NOT BEGIN this section without first recognizing, appreciating, and applauding every single professional and support staff within American healthcare. Once you've lived in the hospital-based system, ridden ambulances, visited patients' homes, you really get to see the strength, courage, resilience, commitment, and empathy of the people who work hard each day to hold a broken system together. My gratitude and appreciation for every one of those people is boundless—from the folks who keep the rooms clean to the transport folks; to the technicians; to the nurses, PAs, and doctors; to all of the support staff; and to the administrators and executives who do their best in a challenging and confusing system. It's not enough, but I want to take this opportunity to say thank you. Know that I and we appreciate you—the smiles, the encouraging words, the kindness, and the enormous professionalism, expertise, and skill you bring. You save lives in more ways than you might imagine. I know that it's easy to forget that as you wake up each morning and just do your job.

Speaking of the professionals who wake up each morning and just do their jobs, I'd like to thank my wife, Lisa, who is one of the most impressive people I've ever met. She is an infectious disease physician and a quality and safety officer in one of the largest healthcare systems in the country. During the COVID-19 pandemic, I and so many others witnessed the awesome expertise that she and her colleagues brought to bear on the deadliest couple of years we've known in our lifetimes. While many of us were sheltering in our homes, she left every morning to work in the hospital. She returned every night with the deep impression of goggles and protective gear imprinted on her face. The ability she and her colleagues had to keep up with the daily changes in our understanding of that disease was breathtaking and lifesaving. In 2022 she was honored as Physician of the Year at Atrium Health (now a part of Advocate Health). She deserved the recognition, but so did every other physician, provider of care, administrator, and support staff who worked under those incredibly stressful and harsh conditions for months on end.

In addition to being a brilliant and empathetic doctor, as well as a healthcare leader, Lisa is an amazing mother to our two children, Emily and Jacob. She is the best life partner I could ever have hoped for. I will admit that I am sometimes jealous of her brain power and sometimes envious of the huge heart she has. There is no question that she is a role model for me and the kids, and I am grateful for her being a part of my life and for me being a part of hers.

Our children, Emily and Jacob, played an outsized role in this book and in my thinking. They were both teenagers at the time of this writing, which is to say that they were nonstop irreverent and unabashedly unreserved about their opinions. While some of their banter and comments border on intolerable, they've pushed me to think in different ways. I authored the book *Reframing Healthcare* four years ago, but what I've discovered is that having teenagers is a constant lesson in reframing. I am immensely grateful for their uncluttered, agile, and fresh thinking and for their curiosity, integrity, and brutal honesty. They have informed, inspired, and changed me in ways that I probably can't begin to understand. I have hope for the future of humanity because it seems to me that their generation will be better and brighter stewards than their progenitors.

The one thing I've learned in writing this book is that it's an amalgam of what I've learned from the people around me, especially my close friends and colleagues. I felt more like a curator than an author at times—just sharing what my peers were teaching me about healthcare. There are way too many names to list, and I'm not going to risk mentioning some and mistakenly leaving out others. I'm fortunate to have family and close friends who are doctors, nurses, executives, and entrepreneurs in healthcare, and what I've learned from them is sprinkled throughout this entire book. In particular, I'd like to thank my Atrium Health colleagues who I am in awe of. I am wowed each and every day by the brilliant minds and hearts of the people I get to call my teammates. I'd also like to thank the courageous leaders and entrepreneurs that I've had the privilege of speaking with and interviewing over the past few years. There is no doubt in my mind that it has been a lifeline for me to be among the 'beyond the walls' leaders on a regular basis and to be inspired, encouraged, and catalyzed by them. If it weren't for the opportunities within these conversations and interviews to get beyond the walls, I'm not sure what I would have done with my career. I'd like to thank Chas Roades and Dr. Lisa Bielamowicz, the incredible founders of the Gist Healthcare podcast, for giving me the permission to use their graphics in chapter 8. I've been learning from them for years and am an avid listener of their daily podcast and reader of their weekly summary. I'd also like to thank my friends and colleagues who proofread this manuscript and provided their wise and gentle feedback.

Finally, I need to thank two incredible individuals who jumped in during the last few weeks of the book writing process. Thank you,

Jess Greenwood and Anne Wong! You helped me make it to the finish line, and I am forever grateful to you both. As long as it took to get this book written, it would have taken a lot longer without your keen expertise and knowledge in healthcare and your wondrous skills and work ethic.